THE WOMAN'S GUIDE TO
RUNNING

hamlyn

THE WOMAN'S GUIDE TO
RUNNING

motivation·training·nutrition·safety

Liz Yelling

To Alex and Rosemary Stanton, my lifetime coaches, without whose effort, constant giving and inspiring support and guidance I would not have inherited the knowledge shared in this book.

The Publisher would like to thank Liz and Martin Yelling for their invaluable contribution to the book at every stage of preparation.

The Woman's Guide to Running has been produced in association with *Running fitness* magazine.

First published in Great Britain in 2007 by
Hamlyn, a division of Octopus Publishing Group Ltd
2–4 Heron Quays, London E14 4JP

Introduction and chapter introduction text copyright © Liz Yelling
The moral rights of the author have been asserted.

Copyright © Octopus Publishing Group Ltd 2007

Distributed in the United States and Canada by Sterling Publishing Co., Inc.,
387 Park Avenue South, New York, NY 10016–8810

ISBN-13: 978-0-600-61405-0
ISBN-10: 0-600-61405-0

A CIP catalogue record for this book is available from the British Library.

Printed and bound in China

10 9 8 7 6 5 4 3 2 1

Notes
This book is not intended as a substitute for personal medical advice. The reader should consult a physician before taking up any exercise programme. While the advice and information are believed to be accurate and true at the time of going to press, neither the author nor the publisher can accept any legal responsibility or liability for errors or omissions that may be made.

Some of the material in this book has appeared previously in *Body Sculpting* (2004), *Cellulite Solutions* (2003), *Firm Abs Flat Stomach* (2004), *Fitball Workout* (2006), *The Pilates Difference* (2003) and *Vitamins & Minerals* (2003), all also published by Hamlyn.

Contents

The great thing about running as a sport and a lifestyle choice is that it is so versatile. Women of any fitness level can run, just about anywhere and at any time. Running does not have to take much out of your day, it does not require lots of expensive equipment and it is something you can do alone or with friends, depending on how you are feeling. All you really need is a little time and a decent pair of running shoes.

Picture this: you are running effortlessly through a leafy park or a field full of flowers. The breeze is flowing through your hair, the sun kisses your skin, you feel energized and alive. In fact, you are probably firmly rooted to your preferred spot on the sofa, with some uninteresting television programme about to start. You have just got home from a tiring day at work, the children are playing up and the thought of going out for a run is very far from your mind – you can always start tomorrow.

The problem is that instead of focusing on how running would improve their lives, if only they would just get out there, many women worry about what will happen when they start running. Everyone will be looking at me, won't they? What would I wear? Will I get out of breath? Will I be fit enough? This book aims to answer all these questions and to show you how to start running – and how to keep going. If you've never run before or if you've run but are stuck in a rut; if you're a regular runner who wants to become a racer or you're a racer who wants to go faster, then this is the book for you.

Why use this book?

As a professional athlete, I know that running is a health-enhancing activity that's within the reach of everybody – and *every body*. This book is designed to be your running 'toolbox', containing everything you need to achieve your health, fitness and running goals. Whatever you want to achieve – your first tentative steps; running 30 minutes without stopping; completing a running event; training for a half-marathon or marathon – this book will guide, support and advise you right the way through your journey. It will prepare you for running today, tomorrow and in the future.

Introduction

You would love to improve your health, to be fitter, to have a slim, toned body, to feel good about yourself. You want to have a positive outlook on life, to be empowered, motivated and inspired. You would like to seek out challenges, meet new people and visit fresh places. Welcome to the world of being a woman runner, for running can – and will – bring all of these benefits, and so much more.

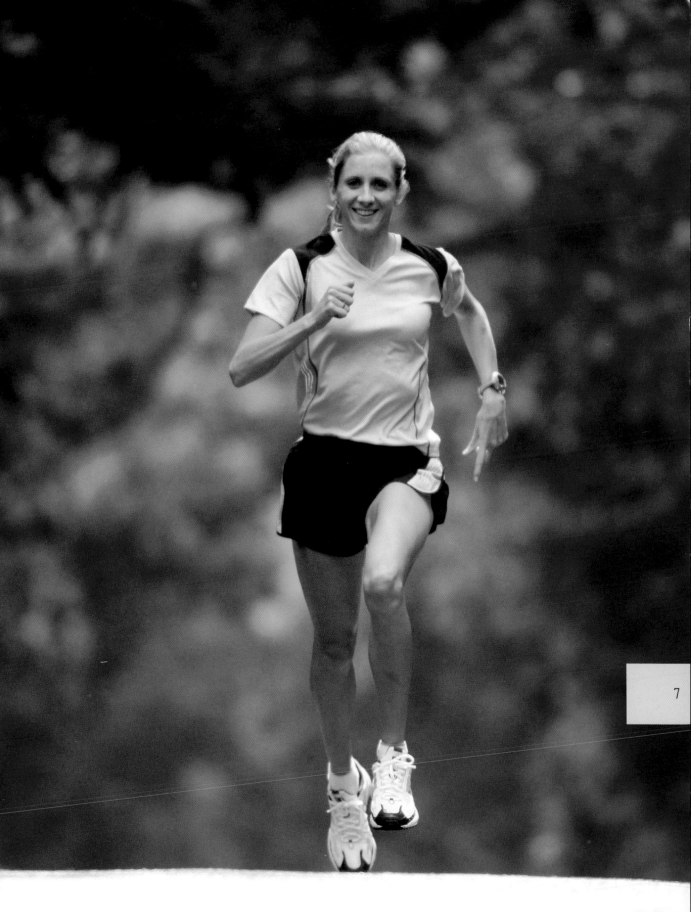

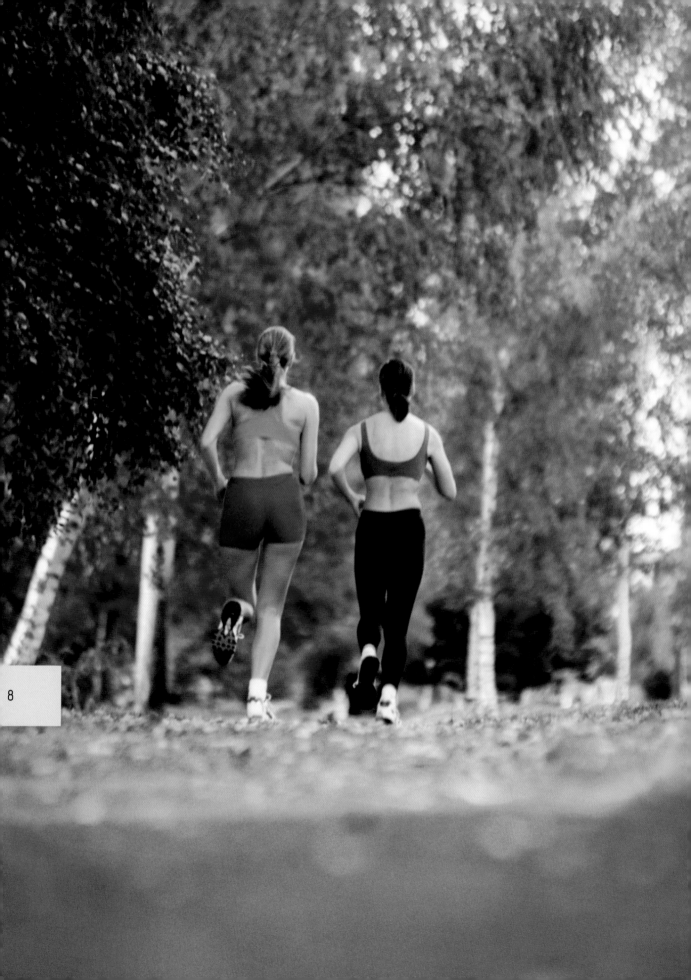

This book wholly recognizes the needs of women runners. It is packed with practical and motivational tips for making your running easier to accomplish, rewarding and enjoyable. It aims to empower you as a woman runner and to equip you with knowledge about every aspect of running, from buying a good pair of women's running shoes to combating premenstrual fatigue and working through a training schedule for a competitive event. Knowledge inevitably brings confidence, so you will be both a confident and competent runner, and as a woman runner you really will experience that liberating feeling of being in control of your body.

Ready, steady, go!

The book is organized into three sections. The first, 'Ready', will get you raring to go by explaining all the wonderful benefits that running will bring, from good health and weight loss to glowing skin and a positive outlook on life. It shows how running can be fitted into even the busiest life and gives some useful time-management ideas as well as all the information you'll need about where and when to run, what to wear and how to choose the right shoes. Diet is inextricably linked to a health-enhancing fitness programme, so this section also examines the importance of a balanced and nutritious diet, with advice that will help you look after your body inside and out.

'Steady' will get you running in a gentle, non-threatening, non-humiliating way. It describes what to expect right from the start, what to do on your first runs and how to improve progressively. All aspects of running training are covered, from the best way to move and breathe to warming up and cooling down. In addition to learning how to run properly, you will also discover how to listen to your body so that you know when not to run – in certain cases of illness or injury. There is also advice about running during pregnancy.

The final section, 'Go!', gives you the confidence to stretch your running boundaries and actively search out running events to participate in. You will discover how to decide which events are right for you, how to enter and what to expect on the day. There are also detailed, comprehensive and practical training schedules for four different sorts of event – 5 km (3.1 miles), 10 km (6.2 miles), half-marathon and marathon. In each case there is a schedule for beginners, improvers and more competent runners, ensuring that runners of all abilities will be able to achieve their goals. Who knows where your running will take you? What I do know is that this book will aid you on your running journey, making the paths you choose easier to follow, safe, enjoyable and inspiring. There is nothing stopping you!

Liz Yelling

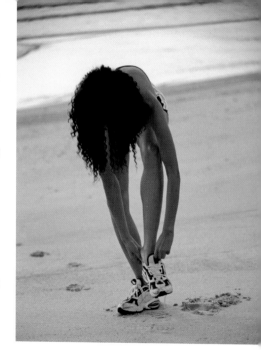

9

EADY...STEADY...

.GO!.....READY...

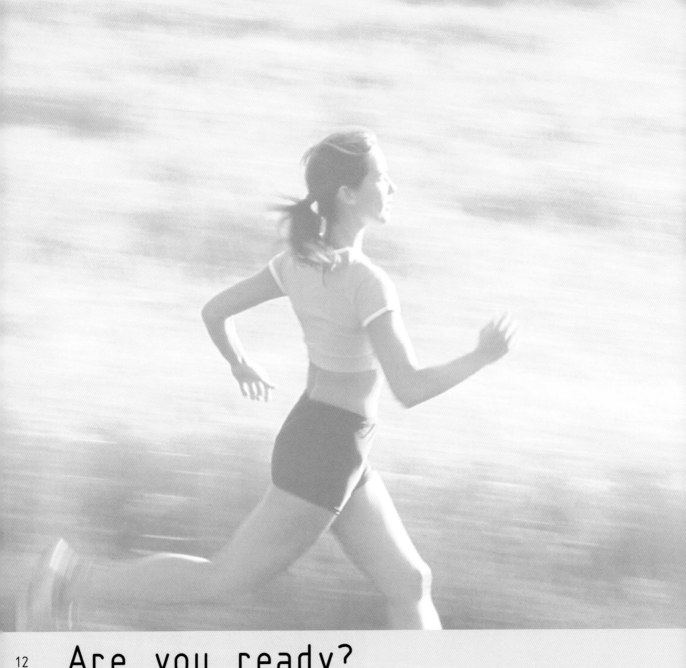

Are you ready?

12

One of the brilliant things about running and being a runner is just how easily it can be slotted into your everyday life. You don't need a huge array of fancy kit, your equipment won't take up half the space in your car and you only need a small amount of time in your day to participate.

So what's the problem? For many women the greatest hurdle is making that commitment, taking those first steps out the front door. You may be ready to start mentally, but do you know how to start physically? Don't panic! Before you even leave the house, there is plenty you can do to prepare yourself for your journey from beginner to regular runner, or from regular runner to expert runner. The following pages contain all you need to know for a push in the right direction.

Deciding why you want to run is a good place to start. This section outlines the tremendous physical benefits of regular running – such as improved general health and reduced risk of a number of medical conditions, including osteoporosis and cardiovascular disease – and it also describes the psychological rewards that becoming a runner will bring. There are many suggestions about where you can run, including ideas for road and off-road running, and invaluable tips on staying safe wherever you choose to run. You'll also find lots of advice about how to make space in your weekly schedule for regular running sessions.

Finding out what to wear before you head out to the shops can save you time and money. Buying a limited number of the right clothes is key, so have a look at the lists of ideal running kit for summer and winter months, as well as the guidance about gadgets such as stopwatches, heart-rate monitors and hydration systems. The most important purchase will, of course, be your shoes and you should read the essential advice on buying the right footwear before making any hasty decisions.

Finally, this section takes a close look at what you should be eating and drinking to provide you with all the nutrition and hydration you need as a woman runner. The focus is on consuming a healthy, balanced daily diet, but there is also key information about the role played by carbohydrates in a runner's diet and the importance of monitoring fluid intake when you exercise. If keeping weight down is one of your running goals, don't forget that a healthy diet is a vital part of the process.

Liz says: 'Don't be daunted by the prospect of becoming a runner. Just get out and try it. Once you've put one foot in front of the other, been out of breath and enjoyed the fresh air, you can call yourself a runner!'

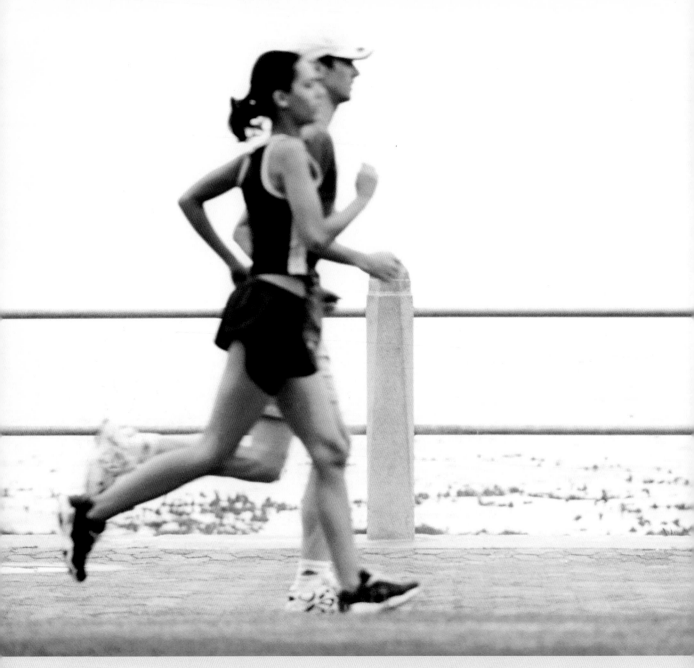

Why running is good for you

Participation in regular physical activity is good for you in many different ways. In the simplest terms, daily moderate activity that might include running two to three times a week will help you manage and maintain a good weight and general good health. Becoming an active person is a lifestyle choice that really will make a difference to your quality of life – and by picking up this book you have already made a start.

Running is one of the easiest sports to take up and make part of your routine. It requires hardly any equipment or pre-planning, and even when the idea of going for a run least appeals – when it's raining or after a challenging day – the minute you take those first tough steps, you will see things differently. Running is fun, rewarding, stimulating, non-humiliating and non-threatening, and will inspire you to achieve things you previously thought impossible.

Health benefits of running

Frequent, health-enhancing exercise has been shown to reduce significantly the risk of suffering from various chronic medical conditions and causes of ill-health, in particular: cardiovascular disease, heart attacks, strokes, obesity, diabetes, hypertension (high blood pressure), arthritis and some cancers. One of the most straightforward, convenient and accessible ways to enjoy regular physical activity is to run.

As well as reducing the risk of primary causes of ill-health, running helps improve and maintain your general health and is a fantastic way to lose and control body weight, to increase muscle strength, flexibility and joint mobility and to improve the condition of your skin. Running really does make you look and feel better; it gives you that 'feel-good factor' and makes you glow!

Additional benefits

Running also provides psychological, emotional and social benefits. You will find that being a runner improves your mental attitude, increases your self-esteem and boosts your confidence. At the same time, it reduces anxiety and depression. Running alone can be a great 'de-stresser', allowing you time to think, or to escape and empty your mind.

Furthermore, running brings with it a great opportunity to meet other women runners, develop friendships and discover new places. Running with friends is not only sociable but can be very motivating, and is a wonderful way of getting started and staying involved – it is harder to find excuses if someone else is relying on your company.

Running can:

- *Boost your immune system*
- *Reduce muscle tension*
- *Help you sleep well*
- *Improve posture*
- *Prevent joint and muscle injury*
- *Help ward off osteoporosis*
- *Reduce cholesterol levels*

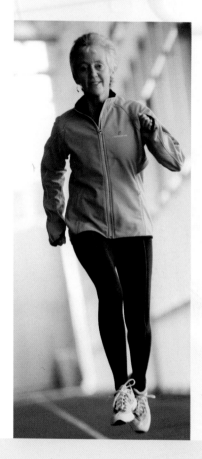

Liz says: 'Being committed to some regular physical activity means you are committed to good health and looking after your body.'

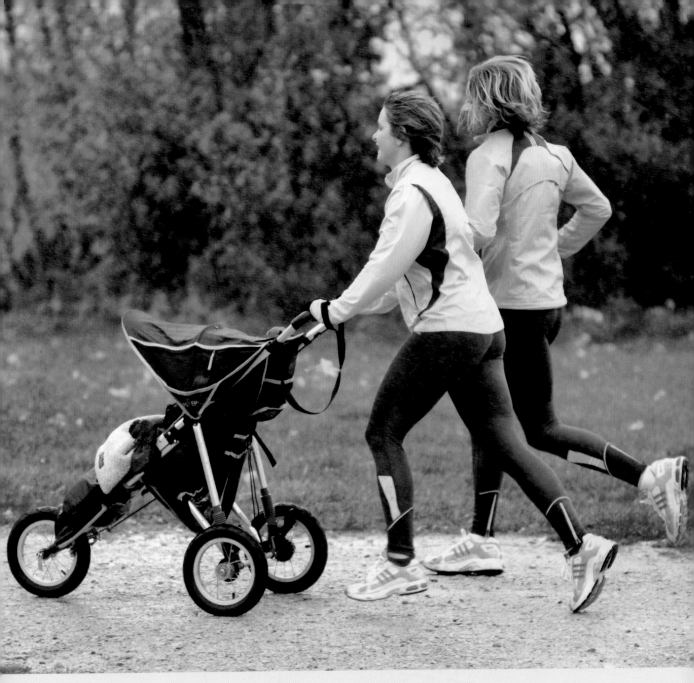

When to run

The key to successful running is knowing when to run. Although this can be any time of day – 8 am in the morning or 7 pm at night – it is important to establish a regular pattern. Develop a running routine and try to stick to it.

Creating balance in your life

The majority of women have busy work-family-life schedules, and fitting everything they would like to do into an everyday pattern is not always straightforward or easy. The thought of adding a run to an already overbooked day might be a chilling one, but once you make the commitment – once you create the time to run – you will never look back.

Going for that run will reward you with valuable 'me time'. It will revitalize and refresh you, helping you to continue juggling the rest of your daily tasks. Creating balance in your life is about acknowledging the things that are important to you, making choices and prioritizing. It's about balancing the things you have to do with the things you want to do. Invariably, your freedom to make choices about your lifestyle will be constrained by other important demands on your time and energy: family, job, available finances. Striking a balance can be problematic, but it isn't impossible.

Of course, every woman's situation is unique, but you will be able to go a long way towards achieving the life you want by taking control of the things you can change and managing those that you cannot. By choosing to acknowledge the importance of your long-term health by becoming a runner, you are accepting responsibility for creating time to run in your day, however busy your schedule.

Time-efficient running

You will be surprised at how easily regular running sessions can be fitted into a busy life. There are various strategies that you can use to make the most of your time. Try running early, before you do anything else – it will raise your metabolic rate and get you ready for the day. Or you could run straight after work, to avoid being interrupted by things waiting to be done at home. Perhaps you could run home from work, or stop on the way for a run that will invigorate and refresh you. An alternative strategy would be to structure your day so that you can run just before you eat lunch.

Top training tips

Strategies for making time:

- *Prioritize. Decide what is important and spend quality time doing it.*
- *Don't feel guilty about going for a run.*
- *Create boundaries around your running time – and keep to them.*
- *Develop a support network. Join a running club, get a running 'buddy', involve your partner and children.*
- *Be creative about your daily schedule and keep a calendar visible to your whole family.*
- *Be flexible. If things don't go to plan, adjust and move on.*
- *Be committed to your running – remember why you do it.*

Liz says: 'You cannot make six minutes out of five just because you manage your time effectively. Each day you are given a new 24 hours. Make the best possible use of this time and don't let it slip through your fingers.'

Top training tips

Great time-savers:

- *Don't procrastinate – just get out there and do it.*
- *Know your route before you head out of the door.*
- *Always keep your running kit in the same place so that you know exactly where to find it.*
- *If you run early, prepare your kit the night before so that it's ready to wear in the morning.*

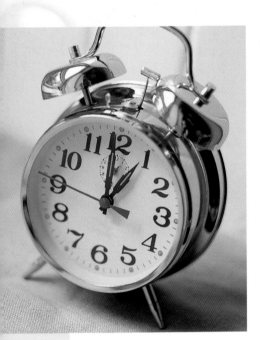

How long to run for

You don't require much time in the day to run. Beginners need to start slowly and progressively, so runs should be short in the early days. As a 'newby' runner, training will take you between 15 and 40 minutes each time. With regular running, your body will become fitter and stronger and you will be able to run for longer.

Initially, try to plan for between three and five exercise sessions a week, allowing a little extra time for changing and showering. Even if you find it hard at first to accommodate exercise in your weekly schedule, you will be amazed at what you can fit into a short amount of time once you have established an effective routine. When you become a real running expert, you can expect to increase to an hour or more per session, by which time you will be adept at saving time: you'll have the right kit to hand, know exactly where you are going to run and be practised in taking a quick shower.

There are no rules stating how long to exercise for: it is all down to personal circumstances, motivation, fitness levels and goals. Remember that a little running is better than no running, even if at first you can only manage a 10 minute walk-run a few times a week. It takes time to become a runner and it is sensible to walk before you can run. In fact, when you first become a runner, it is likely that your first steps will actually be walking (see the beginners' schedules on pages 79 and 81–82). But with patience, motivation and determination, it will not be long before you get into your stride and can run continuously for increasing lengths of time.

Confidence booster

Remember, everyone feels nervous when they start something for the first time. Relish the personal challenge that awaits you. You can do it!

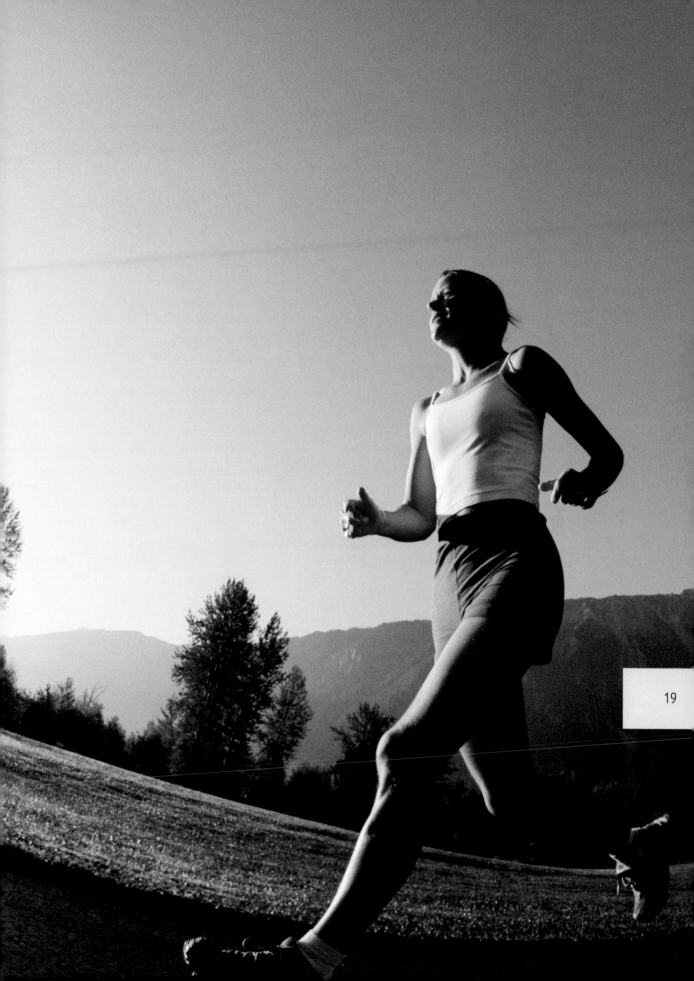

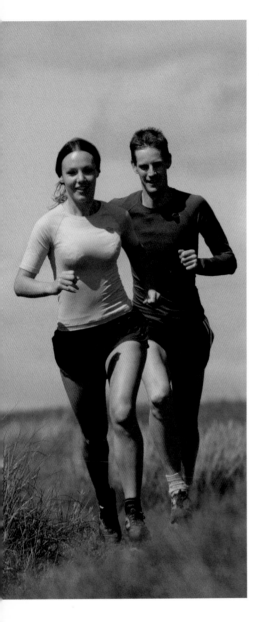

Road running

There are different types of road running. Running in built-up urban areas often means sticking to the pavement or designated footpaths. Choosing a route that does not run alongside major traffic is the best option, as high levels of traffic inevitably bring noise, pollution and congestion. Consider pedestrian traffic, too. It is not a good idea to run through your town at peak times, when you will spend more time dodging and waiting than actually running. An urban park is a great alternative. Many cities and towns have parks that are big enough to run in, with a network of trails and paths.

Minor roads in the country offer the chance to get away from traffic and can be worth a short drive to find them. These roads don't usually have pavements, so it is vital to stay alert and run close to the edge of the road, against the flow of any traffic. Avoid blind bends by moving across the road at a safe and suitable point. Country-road running gives you the opportunity to enjoy relatively quiet running and country views.

Off-road running

For totally traffic-free running, and to experience the real thrills of running 'away from it all', try getting off-road. There are numerous options to choose from, depending on where you live. It might take a little time and research to find the best off-road running, but the effort will be well worth it. Lakes frequently have easy-to-follow trails around the perimeter; coastal paths can provide rugged cliff-top runs with spectacular ocean scenery; disused railways are brilliant for flat running, as are canal towpaths and riverside walks; mountain trails can be challenging but rewarding, with breathtaking views.

Many country areas have designated and waymarked footpaths and trails that run across fields and through forests and parkland. Some regions, in particular National Parks, have official long-distance walking and hiking paths that are also perfect for running. The wonderful thing about running in open spaces is that you really get to soak up the beauty of your surroundings and appreciate the wildlife and the landscape.

Where to run

Many women begin running on the treadmill at the local gym and are not sure how or where to progress. The gym treadmill offers a safe, controlled and convenient environment for your workout, but lacks the stimulation that running in the great outdoors can provide. Don't be afraid to take steps away from the treadmill and turn your running into a whole new vibrant and exciting exercise experience.

It is a good idea to have several pairs of trainers (for example, a pair of trail shoes and a pair of supportive road runners) and wear them for different runs. This will ensure that you don't always run in the same shoes. You could always buy two pairs of the same type if you discover a brand and model that suit you particularly well.

Seeking professional help

Visit a reputable specialist running or triathlon retailer, taking a pair of your old shoes with you. An assistant will examine the shoes to see how they have worn, and also look at your feet and ask questions about any past or present injuries and your training, before suggesting a shortlist of shoes for you to try on. Some shops use specialist equipment to measure the force with which your foot strikes the ground.

Buying running shoes

- Find your old running/sports shoes and stand them on a table with the back/heel facing you.
- Imagine a line running from the top of the heel tab down to the bottom of the shoe and look at how the upper is warped where it joins the mid-sole. If the upper leans inwards, then you over-pronate. If it leans outwards, you under-pronate. If the upper is not distorted, then you are a neutral runner. It is worth noting that most people over-pronate.
- If you over-pronate, you need support shoes, which offer both cushioning and support along the inside (medial side) of the mid-sole to stop your feet rolling over too far. Runners who are heavier, or who over-pronate severely, may need motion-control shoes. These are more supportive and are designed to cope with greater over-pronating loads being placed on the shoe. If you under-pronate or have neutral feet, you need neutral, also called cushioning, shoes.
- If using the shoe primarily for on-road use, choose a support or neutral shoe. Look for good cushioning in the heel and also in the forefoot – particularly if your forefoot hits the ground first when you run. The upper should fit well and it should be snug around the heel and mid-foot, but more roomy in the toe box. You also want good flexibility under the ball of the foot to allow your foot to move naturally.
- Your shoe should also provide adequate grip. If you require shoes predominantly for off-road use, consider buying a pair of trail shoes. Look for good grip from a lugged outsole, a supportive, snug and durable upper and adequate cushioning for the terrain.
- Don't be afraid to ask to take your running shoes for a walk or jog up the road from the shop. A high-quality specialist retailer will let you do this.

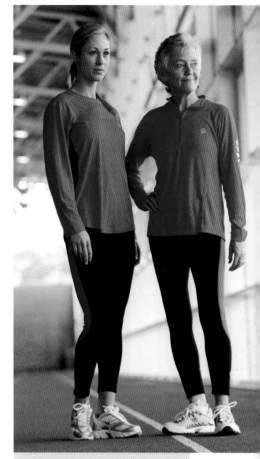

Safety first

Always wear the right clothing for the conditions and terrain you are running in, and avoid inappropriately revealing items.

Use your heart rate as a tool to guide your training, but don't become a slave to it. Instead, try basing your effort on how you feel. If you feel like trying hard, run quickly; if you think you need a break, and just want to enjoy the fresh air, then run slowly.

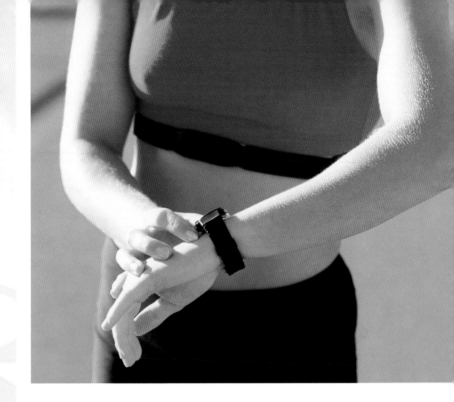

Stopwatches

A good stopwatch is an invaluable piece of equipment for a runner. Most stopwatches have a clear display showing your total running time and are also able to record split and lap times – which will be useful when you start to run specific training sessions.

Heart-rate monitors

Consisting of a chest strap (the 'transmitter') and wristwatch (the 'receiver'), a heart-rate monitor can be a great aid to your running. This piece of kit is worth investing in, particularly if you are a beginner, as it reads the number of beats made by the heart in one minute (as beats per minute or BPM, see page 49), letting you know precisely how much effort you are putting in. As you exercise, your heart is required to pump faster in order to circulate more blood around

What to carry

Safety first

Remember that heart rates are highly individual. Compare your own responses from day to day, but don't make comparisons with the heart rates of other runners.

your body; the harder you exercise, the faster your heart will beat. Once you have been running regularly for a while, you will find it easier to recognize the patterns of your heart rate, and be able to adjust your effort accordingly to make the most of your training.

Heart-rate monitors come in all sorts of guises and have a range of different functions. Some measure speed and distance at the same time, showing you how fast and far you are going. Others can download information onto your computer so that you can plot improvement over time. More basic – and cheaper – models simply offer a visual display of your heart-rate reading as you run. What you buy depends on how technically minded you are, how much time you want to spend analysing your runs and how much money you want to lay out. It is advisable to start with something simple.

Water bottles and hydration systems

It is essential to drink before, during and after exercise (see 'What to drink', pages 34–35). Bottles of sports drinks are ideal for taking in your kit bag or carrying on your runs. Drinking while you are out running can be tricky, but there are products designed to help. Small hand-held drinks bottles carry enough fluids for a short run. 'Camelbacks', 'fuel belts', water belts and other hydration systems are designed for wearing around your waist or carrying on your back. They are like very small rucksacks, either with space for slotting in drinks bottles or with a removable reservoir ('bladder') that can be filled. All reusable bottles and bladders must be kept clean with the same kind of sterilizing solution used for soaking babies' bottles. (See also page 122 for information on marathon hydration.)

Kit bags and rucksacks

Good-quality kit bags come in all shapes and sizes and are useful for transporting your running clothes and generally keeping yourself well organized. A special running rucksack is a sensible idea if you need to be mobile with your kit.

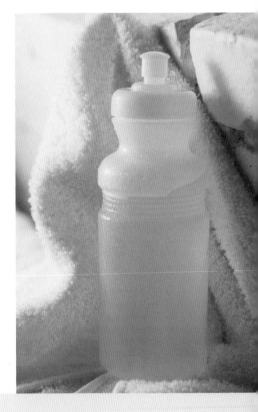

Liz says: 'It can be a great stress-reliever not to clock-watch. Once in a while, just get out and run for however long you fancy and at whatever pace you like.'

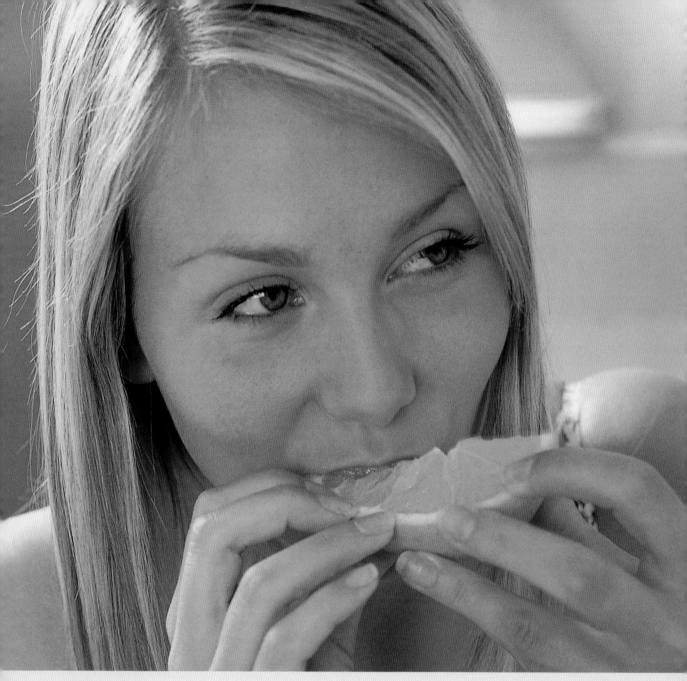

What to eat

Healthy eating is not complicated. A balanced diet that includes plenty of fresh produce is
a real essential for any woman who wants her body to work to the best of its potential.
To complement your running, you need to focus on eating the right things at the right
times, even if you have introduced running as part of a weight-loss programme.

Running is something that all women can do, and do well. To be a successful runner does not mean running faster than anyone else. It means being able to run at your own controlled pace, with confidence, balance, rhythm, posture and style, on a variety of terrains and for a sustained, but varied, amount of time. There is no single route to success – it comes in different forms. A real achiever may be someone who has just completed her first-ever 15 minute non-stop run or 12 week running programme, or who has carved minutes off her personal best times. It may be a woman who has run every day for a year, or who runs with a terminal illness, or who raises money for charity. The possibilities are endless. Above all, being a good runner means that you run regularly, that you stick to your training plan, that you strive to meet the targets you set for yourself and, essentially, that you enjoy it.

Good running form

There is more to running, technically, than simply putting one foot in front of the other. Some runners seem to flow effortlessly, oozing efficiency, speed and style, while others seem to be ungainly and waste energy. Some runners have a long stride, others a short one; some lift their knees very high, while others have almost no pick-up at all.

A stylish, effective and relaxed running style can be learned and will make you economical and smooth in your stride and breathing. It will also help to prevent running-related injuries. Create balance in your form by following a few fundamental technique guidelines:

- **Head:** Aim to keep your head still, steady and facing forwards. Keep your eyes looking a few steps in front of you, studying the terrain under your feet with occasional downward glances.
- **Shoulders:** Keep your shoulders relaxed and hanging naturally. Don't hunch upwards or allow your shoulders to rotate unnecessarily.
- **Arms:** A good arm action counterbalances the forces generated by your legs. Your arms should be held bent at about 90 degrees by your side.

Confidence booster

Running is all about finding balance. If you have balance you will flow, feel capable and confident, recover quickly and be willing to push boundaries. Without balance you will feel unmotivated, lethargic and heavy. Injury and illness can upset your running balance, as can an inadequate diet, stress and emotional upset. A short run can really help by putting things in perspective, but don't forget that you can also skip a run if other priorities take over.

Liz says: 'Becoming a successful runner takes a mixture of patience and persistence; it does not happen overnight. You will experience highs and lows on your journey – enjoy the highs; accept and learn from the lows.'

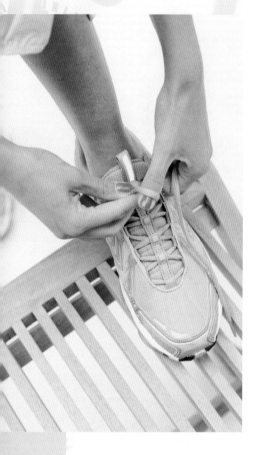

Don't bring them all the way across your body as you run, but allow them to move forwards and backwards close to your body, alternating opposite arm with opposite leg. Each should swing like a pendulum naturally by your side, with the elbow coming up behind you and the hand raised in front.

- **Hands:** Hold each hand comfortably in a light fist; don't clench your fingers tightly. Keep each hand below the level of your shoulder as you bring it forwards with each arm swing. Your hand and forearm will naturally come slightly across your body.
- **Torso:** Your chest should be facing the direction of travel. Try to avoid twisting your midsection from side to side. Avoid leaning too far forwards or leaning backwards. Keep your body upright and your trunk and pelvis stable and balanced.
- **Hips:** Keep each hip facing the direction of travel and keep it 'high'. Your hips should be extended, pushing your body forwards and upwards.
- **Knees:** Drive your knees forwards in opposition to your arms. They should come up to around hip height in front of you (the faster you run, the higher your knee and hip drive). Avoid running with a knee lift that is very low – you will 'shuffle' as a result – or too high. Your knees, hips and lower legs should be kept in a lateral line.
- **Lower legs and ankles:** These will naturally follow the drive of your knee and hip. Bring the lower leg forwards and down, allowing the foot to contact the ground. Keep your ankles flexible and allow them to relax.
- **Feet and footstrike:** A smooth, rolling action from heel to mid-foot to toe is effective for regular road running. Try to avoid 'slapping' the ground with your foot. The faster you run, the more you drive upwards, using the balls of your feet and toes. The foot can roll outwards and inwards as it contacts the ground. This rolling action is known as supination or pronation (see 'The right footwear', pages 24–25).

How to breathe

Your breathing rate adjusts itself automatically all the time, increasing when you walk upstairs quickly, climb a hill or run for the bus, and slowing down when you are resting or asleep. This is a natural response to your body's need to take in and distribute oxygen. Being out of breath – something you will certainly experience as a runner – is perfectly normal and nothing to worry about. Embrace breathlessness as you learn to recognize, manage and extend your physical boundaries. The more running you do, the easier your breathing will become.

When you exercise, you need to take deeper breaths and breathe more often to provide the extra oxygen your body needs. If you are relaxed when you run, your breathing patterns will adjust automatically. It does not matter if you inhale or exhale through your mouth or nose, or both – do whatever feels the most comfortable and the most natural (although the mouth may work best, as it allows more air to pass through). You will soon discover that your breathing rates change according to your level of fitness, the type of running you are doing and the terrain (see 'Types of running training', pages 60–63).

running programme will take place over a number of weeks and months. To a certain extent, progression happens naturally as you become fitter, stronger and more used to running. The key is to avoid increasing the frequency and duration of your workouts at the same time as you increase their intensity.

3. Specificity

Of course, the best way to improve your running is to run, but you should also spend time on complementary activities. Other cardiovascular exercise, such as cycling and swimming, will help boost your fitness and benefit your running. The principle of specificity is particularly important when it comes to event training. If you aim to run a marathon, for example, you'll need to train specifically for the particular challenges of that event.

4. Reversibility

If you don't run with relative frequency (at least twice a week), you will start to lose the running fitness you have developed. Furthermore, it takes less time to lose that fitness than it does to build it up. It does not matter if you miss a few runs – say owing to injury or illness – but if it becomes habitual, you will see your fitness and running ability drop. Don't rush back into training after some time off, but let your body adapt and regain your fitness progressively.

5. Recovery

Linked to progression and overload, this is probably the most crucial, yet most neglected, training principle. When you train you give a shock to your system, after which your body rebuilds itself stronger. But this can only happen if you allow your body enough recovery time. It is important to remember that if you simply increase the distance, speed and frequency of your runs, without regular rest and appropriate recovery strategies, then your body will be at risk of illness and injury. As you progress, your definition of recovery will change, and any good training schedule will build in regular recovery as an essential component of the programme.

Great recovery strategies

- *Bananas are brilliant recovery foods. Eat one within 15 to 30 minutes of running.*
- *Drink plenty of fluids. It takes longer to recover if you are not fully hydrated.*
- *To help the circulation in your legs, wear tight training tights or flight socks if you have a 30 minute or longer drive home after training.*

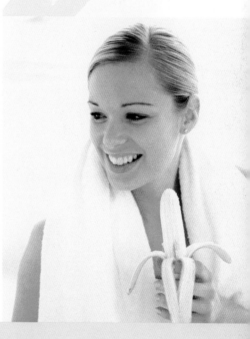

Liz says: 'Don't be too ambitious on your first attempts. You must allow for a few weeks of improvement. Just add a little every week and before you know it you'll be up and running.'

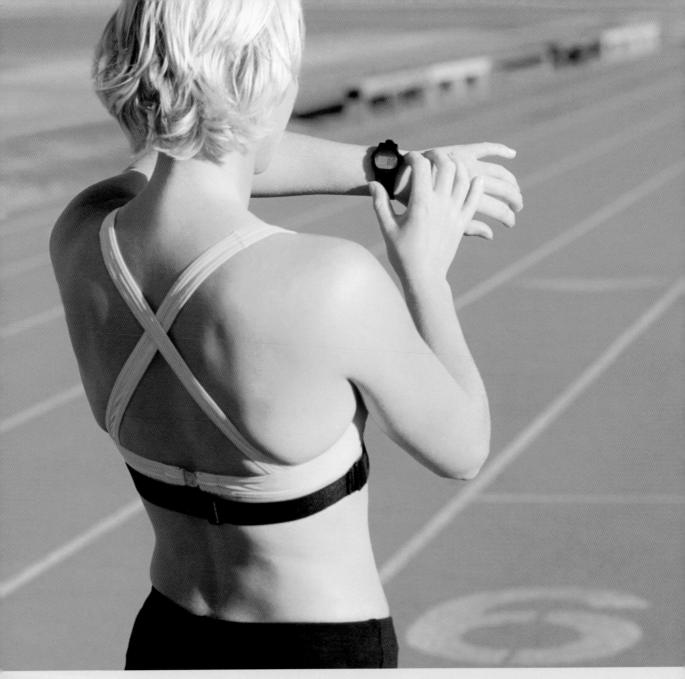

Physical effects of running

Your body responds to exercise in a variety of different ways. In simple terms, these can be considered as immediate, short-term and longer-term effects. You will probably find that you have some initial aches and pains to overcome before you can enjoy the many physical benefits that running will bring.

Immediate effects

The first physical changes you will notice occur the moment you start running. Your breathing rate increases, your heart rate goes up, you experience a rise in your body temperature and an aching sensation in your leg muscles and you may also feel thirsty.

- **Changes to breathing rate:** As you break into your stride, you will need to take more frequent and deeper breaths. If you are not used to running, you can control breathlessness by starting with walk-runs. As you continue to exercise, your ability to run without getting out of breath will soon increase.
- **Increased heart rate:** It is perfectly normal to feel your heart rate go up when you start to exercise, and for it to stay elevated during exercise. You can use a heart-rate monitor to help you measure your responses (see page 26). The average adult resting heart rate is approximately 72 beats per minute (BPM). When you are running hard, you can expect a heart rate in excess of 140 BPM and up to 200 BPM.
- **Rise in temperature:** Like an engine, your body warms up quickly when you run and, within a few minutes, you start to sweat. Sweating is your body's natural cooling mechanism. For this reason, don't be tempted to wear too many layers of clothing when the weather is cold. In summer months and humid conditions, your sweat rate increases even more as your body attempts to keep you cool. It is very important to wear the right clothing for the season (see 'What to wear', pages 22–25) and to keep well hydrated before, during and after exercise (see 'What to drink', pages 34–35).
- **Aching leg muscles:** The major muscles you are using to run may feel uncomfortable. This is only natural, especially when you first start to run. You may experience a burning sensation in your muscles, which will ease if you reduce your pace or walk for a few minutes. With an appropriate, progressive and regular running schedule, the aches and pains you feel initially will soon disappear.

Top training tip

Experiment with your heart rate when you run. Try to feel your heart rate increase and decrease as you vary your pace.

Liz says: 'Once you've started your running programme, don't stop! Your legs may feel sore, but given appropriate recovery periods, your muscles will soon adapt to the new challenges.'

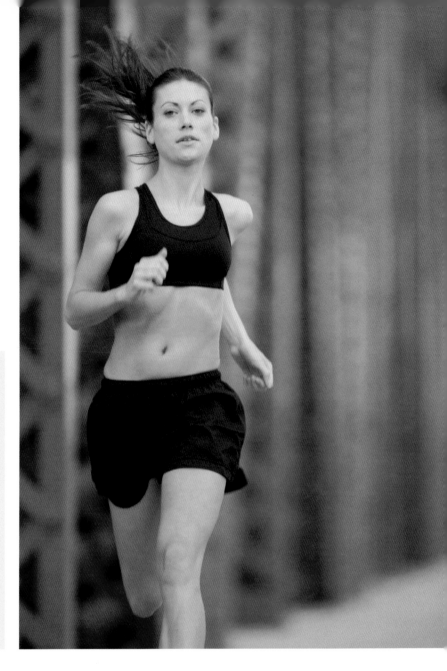

Confidence booster

You will now begin to experience the thrill of calling yourself a runner. When you get back from your first run, knowing you are improving your health and fitness, you will feel invigorated, self-confident and empowered.

Run how you feel

It is possible to use the immediate physical sensations produced by running as a guide to control your effort. A scale of 'perceived exertion', ranging from 6–20, was initially conceived in the 1950s by the Swedish researcher Gunnar Borg. The scale is commonly used by athletes in training to help them run at a particular speed according to the physical effects they are experiencing. In general, the faster you run, the harder it feels and the tougher it is to maintain. Try to reflect on how you feel when you run – using a 1–5 scale, ranging from very easy to very hard – and match these feelings to your heart rate. You will notice that your heart rate is higher when you are more tired, running faster and putting in more effort. Developing an understanding of the connection between your 'ratings of perceived exertion' and your running will help you judge when and how to run fast and when to rest and run easy.

Short-term effects

Because your body is so good at adapting to meet physical challenges, you will find that the more running you do, the easier it gets. These improvements take time, however, and you are likely to face a few hurdles along the way.

- **Aching muscles:** One or two days after starting an exercise programme, you may experience muscle soreness, especially in your legs and hips – particularly if you are new to running. This is quite normal. When you run, you cause minor trauma in your muscles and the soreness is your body's way of recovering and adapting. The aches and pains will ease within a day or so and will be less intense and less frequent each time you run. The key is to follow a progressive programme that allows your muscles to adapt.
- **Reduced energy levels:** In the first few days and weeks of running, you will feel more tired than normal and may need to sleep more. As your body adjusts, you will start to feel refreshed after running and the quality of your sleep patterns will soon improve.
- **Improved health:** A regular exercise routine will bring you physical benefits even from the earliest days. What's more, the knowledge that you're already well on the way to becoming a regular runner will be a great boost to your confidence and self-esteem!

Longer-term effects

The long-term physical gains of regular running are outlined in 'Health benefits of running' (see page 15). After a few weeks of progressive, appropriately structured running, you will start to see the first signs of improvement in your fitness levels. You will notice that you are starting to breathe more easily and with more control throughout your run. Your legs no longer ache during or after your runs, rather you feel 'bouncy' and recover quickly. Your heart does not start to race as soon as you break into your stride, you can run for longer and your usual routes take less time – you are running faster with less effort.

These are the first signals that your body is adapting to regular running – in other words, that your training is working. If your running programme has been married with a healthy, balanced diet, you will also begin to notice a change in your body shape. You will be leaner and lighter, you will see alterations in your muscle definition and tone and your skin complexion will have improved.

Timescale

You will find running starts to become a little easier after two to three weeks, and much easier after six to eight weeks. It takes four to six weeks of regular running before you start to notice any positive changes in your body weight, shape and tone, but these will continue to improve the more you run. After four to six months of regular running, you will be able to really appreciate all the changes that have taken place.

Key adaptations

- *Breathing becomes easier as you start to take in oxygen and utilize it more effectively.*
- *Your heart rate decreases as your heart becomes more efficient at pumping blood.*
- *Your lungs become stronger.*
- *Circulation improves as more tiny blood vessels develop.*
- *Muscles and connective tissues strengthen, allowing you to keep going for longer.*
- *Muscles recover more quickly, ready for each new session.*
- *Your body utilizes food more efficiently, producing increased amounts of energy.*

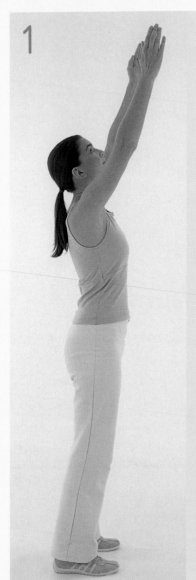
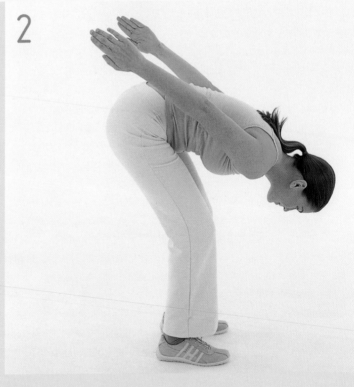

Swing downs

1 Stand tall, with your arms extended above your head and your abdominal and thigh muscles pulled in.

2 Swing your arms down, leaning over and bending your knees as you go. As you swing low, straighten your legs briefly, then bend them again as you swing back to upright. Do 8–10 good strong swings down and up.

Warming up

An effective warm-up is crucial, reducing the risk of soreness or injury and getting you focused and raring to go. As a general rule, include 5–10 minutes of very light aerobic activity, followed by some gentle joint and muscle mobility exercises. Your warm-up will vary depending on your experience and the type of running you are doing. For a total beginner, a warm-up may consist of 5 minutes easy walking. For a more experienced runner, a warm-up may be a 10 or 15 minute jog, with mobility exercises and perhaps some session-specific exercises, too. Take time to prepare your muscles appropriately.

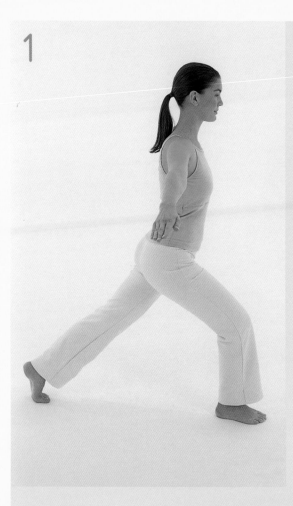

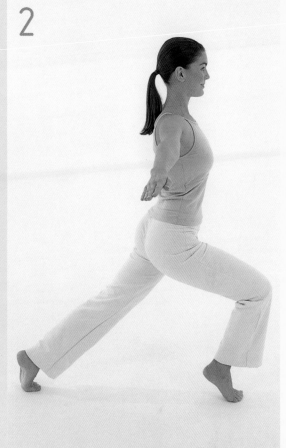

Lunge

1 Place one leg behind you in a lunge position and extend your arms out to the sides. Straighten the back leg, bending the front leg at a right angle and with the heel of your back foot off the floor. Maintain this position for several seconds. The weight of your body should be equally placed between both feet as you hold the position.

2 Lift the heel of your front foot and try to hold this position briefly. Repeat on the other leg.

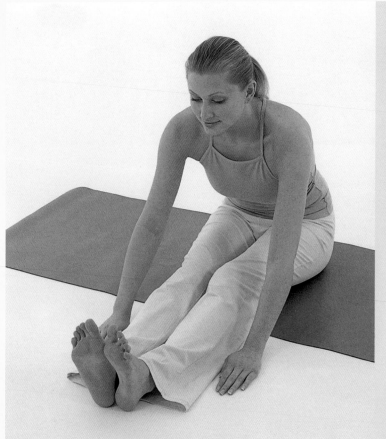

Stretch 1

Sit on the floor as tall as you can with your legs outstretched and feet flexed. Lean forwards and stretch your arms towards your feet. Aim to press forwards from the bottom of your back, to feel the stretch in your back as well as in your hamstrings.

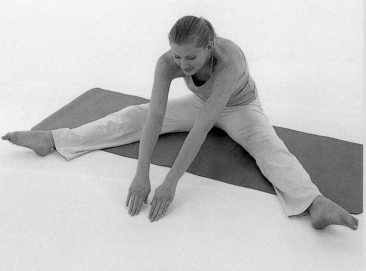

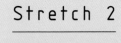

Stretch 2

Sit on the floor with your legs out to the sides and place your hands on the floor in front of you. Gently walk your hands along the floor away from you, pulling your chest towards the floor. You will feel this stretch along your inner thighs and hamstrings. Reach as far as you comfortably can, hold, then walk your hands a little further forwards.

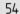

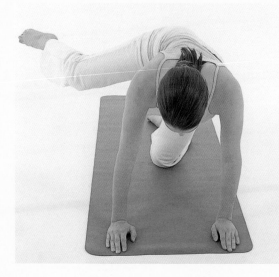

Tabletop

1 Get down on all fours, resting on your hands and knees and keeping your back straight. Lift one leg out to the side, keeping the knee bent and your weight equally balanced on the three remaining limbs.

2 Hold the position, feeling the side of the hip and thigh working, then raise the bent leg slightly higher and lower again in a pulsing movement. Perform 10 repetitions of the lift on first one leg, then the other.

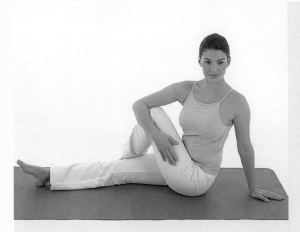

Sit and twist

1 Sit on the floor with your legs outstretched. Bend your left leg up towards your chest, cross it over your right leg and place your left foot flat on the floor.

2 Turn your torso towards the knee and wrap your right arm around the upright leg. Pull the knee into your body, feeling the stretch in the left buttock. Hold for 10–15 seconds, then release. Repeat on the other side.

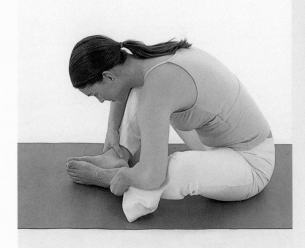

Sit and lean

1 Sit on the floor with your legs outstretched. Bring your feet towards your crotch so that the soles are facing and your legs are bent either side of your body.

2 Hold your ankles and slowly start to lean forwards. Move slowly as you will feel a tightness in the hips. You will also feel the top of the buttocks and lower back start to stretch out. Lean as far as possible, then return to an upright position. Repeat, leaning slightly further the second time.

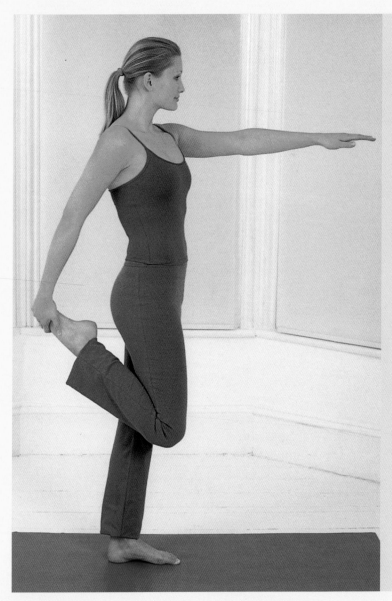

Thigh stretch

1 Stand up straight, then lift your right ankle up behind you, bending your knee. Grasp your foot and gently pull it towards your bottom. You will feel this stretch in your thigh.

2 Hold the position for 30 seconds, using your other arm for balance if you need to.

3 Lower the foot, then repeat with the other leg.

Cooling down

After running, you must give your body time to cool down before you shower. These cooling-down stretches will increase the mobility and elasticity of the different groups of muscles used during running, helping to prevent injuries. Pilates exercises are also very suitable for cooling down (see pages 72–77).

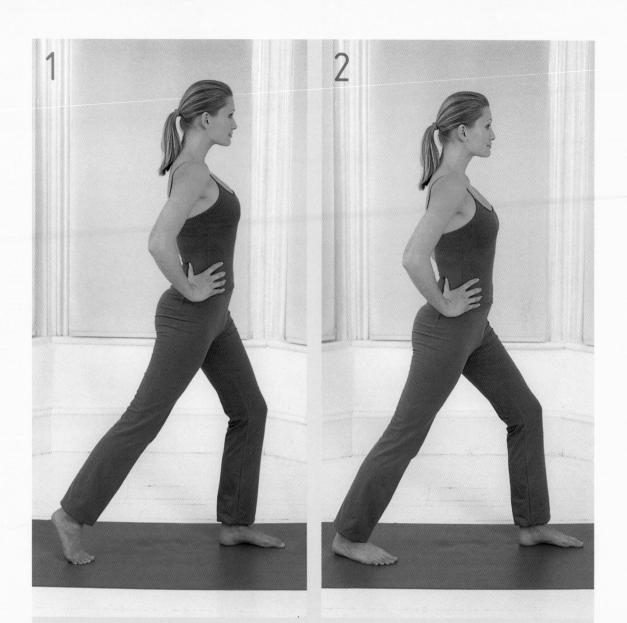

Calf stretch

1 Step forwards with your left leg and bend your knee. Your right leg will straighten and your right heel will come off the floor.

2 Keeping your right leg straight, gently try to push your right heel back down. Hold for 30 seconds when you feel the stretch. Release gently and swap legs.

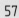

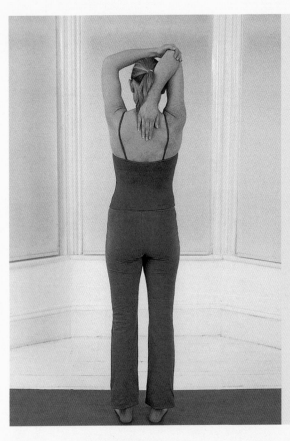

Tricep stretch

1 Reach your hand up and over your shoulder so that your arm is bent, with the elbow pointing upwards and the palm of your hand flat on your back.

2 Using your other arm, gently press the upper arm backwards. Hold for 30 seconds, then swap arms.

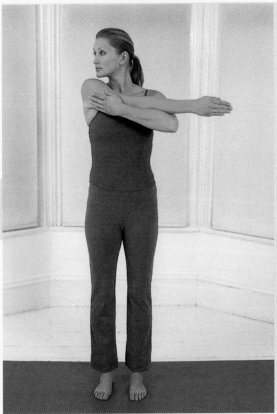

Deltoid stretch

1 Stand up straight and reach your right arm across your body at roughly shoulder height. Use your left arm, placed just above the elbow, to push your right arm gently closer to your body.

2 Hold for 30 seconds, then swap arms.

Hamstring stretch

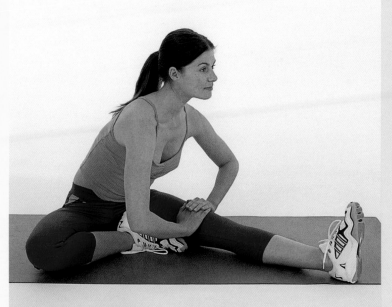

1 Sit on the floor, your left leg outstretched and the other tucked in, your hips square on to the outstretched leg. Straighten your back, lifting your upper body, and then take in a deep breath. As you breathe out, stretch out over the straightened leg, placing hands on thighs with arms bent.

2 Keep the left foot gently flexed and keep the stretching leg as straight as possible – try not to let the back of the knee lift off the ground. Hold for 15–20 seconds and then swap legs.

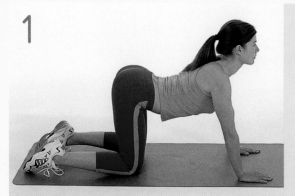

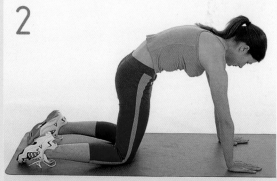

Cat curls

1 Kneel with your hands on the floor, directly under the line of your shoulders, fingers pointing forwards. Your knees should be in line with your hips. Hollow your back, while gently raising your head.

2 Slowly arch your back, vertebra by vertebra, into a hunch while dropping your head. Repeat the movement 10 times, slowly.

Power walking

Power walking is the best way to start your running programme if you are a total beginner. It allows you to become used to exercise and starts to get your heart, lungs and muscles working.

The technique of power walking is perhaps best described as reaching a maximum speed without lifting both feet off the ground at one time. Your stride should be slightly longer than your normal walking stride and your posture should be upright but relaxed. Get into a nice smooth rhythm. Keep your head up and your eyes forwards. Swing one arm, bent at a 90 degree angle, so that your hand comes to approximately shoulder height in front of you. Swing the other arm, again at a 90 degree angle, backwards until your thumb reaches your hip pocket so that the elbow is in unison with the hand in front of you. The intensity of the walk is determined by your arms, not your legs, so swing your arms to the speed you would like your legs to move.

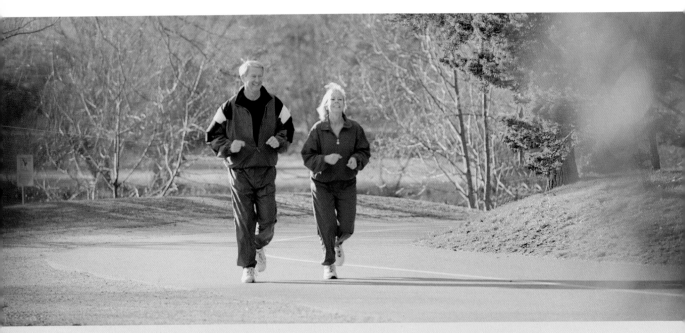

Types of running training

There are a variety of different ways in which you can run, and the type of running you do will depend on your level of experience, your fitness, the stage you are at in your running programme and the reasons you run. When you start training, the majority of your runs will be easy walk-runs, light jogging and steady runs. However, as you progress and get stronger and faster, you will also want to try different running methods.

Walk-run

This type of running training is ideal for beginners, allowing you to build up your running progressively at a level that suits your ability and fitness. It is a good basic aerobic workout that benefits your cardiovascular system, preparing it for the running to come.

The technique is simply a combination of paced walking interspersed with light jogging. The amount of time you spend walking and jogging can and should vary. As you get fitter, you will spend more time jogging and less time walking. Use landmarks such as lampposts, street corners, road junctions and trees as targets to jog to or walk between.

Easy runs

An easy run is a slow run or jog and it is the natural progression from the walk-run introduction. This type of running will further develop your cardio-respiratory and cardiovascular systems (heart, lungs and circulation), and improve muscle strength. As a beginner, many of your first runs will be easy runs, but as you improve you will want to – and will need to if you wish to go faster – include more challenging runs in your workouts.

Easy runs are also brilliant for active recovery – that is, when you feel the need for a break from some of your harder, faster running. They also suit days when you feel tired or lacking in motivation.

Steady runs

Steady runs teach your body to make the best use of its fuel reserves – they are good calorie burners, strengthen your muscles, ligaments and tendons and encourage your body to become more efficient at taking in and distributing oxygen to the working muscles. Along with tempo runs, intervals, fartleks and hill runs, steady runs will really improve your stroke volume (the amount of blood pumped out per heartbeat) and your cardiac output (the amount of blood pumped around the body per minute). The technique is simple: run at a pace at which you can chat to a friend.

Confidence booster

Remember that you will have both good and bad days. On good days, you will glide through your run, feeling energized, strong and powerful. On bad days, for no apparent reason, your run will be a struggle, everything will ache and time will drag. Fortunately, the good days usually far outnumber the bad ones!

Liz says: 'If you want your running to improve, it is essential to mix different types of running training. Set yourself realistic and challenging targets each time you leave to exercise.'

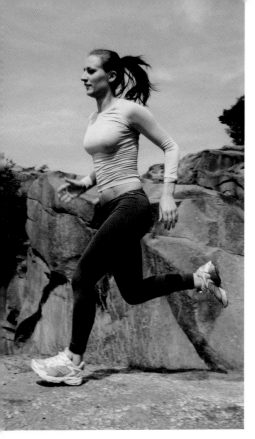

Tempo runs

Running at 'tempo' speed is running at a pace at which you feel on the threshold of comfort. This is great for pushing your limits. You really have to concentrate to keep running and holding a conversation is virtually impossible. As you become more experienced, you will learn how to find your tempo pace, which is likely to change the fitter you get.

Tempo running is the best way to improve the economy of your running – that is, how efficient you are at taking in and utilizing oxygen and at converting stored fuel into energy for exercise. Tempo runs teach your body to adapt to running at a slightly higher intensity than steady running, they develop strength and endurance and burn more calories. Tempo runs are one of the best training methods for racing practice: although not run at race speed, they demand a high level of motivation and concentration to keep going at the desired pace. Tempo running is a crucial aspect of every training schedule.

Long runs

Long runs are usually done at a slow pace and are great for developing stamina and endurance. They help you to concentrate on your running for extended periods – exactly what you need if you are training for a marathon. Prolonged running teaches your body to utilize different sources of stored energy as fuel, as running slower for longer requires fats as fuel in addition to carbohydrates.

A long run means, simply, running for longer than during your other weekly runs. Of course, the duration varies according to level of fitness, running experience, phase of running training programme and the distance (if any) you wish to race. Pace is the key here: because you are running for longer, you will run more slowly. Aim for about 1 minute per 1.6 km (1 mile) slower than you would run during a regular steady run.

Fartlek

Fartlek is a Swedish word for 'speed play'. This method teaches you how to change pace and run at a range of intensities. It overloads the muscles, heart and lungs in a different way to single-paced running and, with time and adaptation, improved fitness and technique are noticeable. Fartlek helps you learn about breathing patterns and incorporating recovery into your running time. It is a good way to build up to interval running (see opposite).

Fartlek is about running fast, running slow, whenever you feel like it! It means mixing easy, steady and fast running for varying times and distances, with differing amounts of recovery. It is best done over varied terrain. For example, you might run hard up one hill and recover as you jog down the other side, or you might run steady to the next lamppost and run easy to another landmark before running hard to the next. Don't worry too much about how long you run for, just ensure that you include noticeable changes in pace. It is a good idea to start with easy and steady running in the first half of your fartlek and build up to fast sections in the second half.

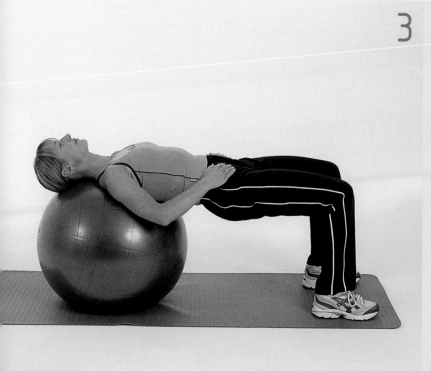

3 Continue to walk away from the ball until your shoulders come to rest on it. Your head and neck should feel comfortable on the ball. With your stomach pulled in and spine in a neutral position, anchor and support your body by using your buttock muscles.

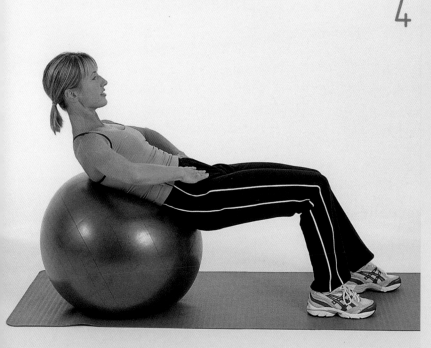

4 To return to the start position, reverse the movement and walk your feet towards the ball. Begin the body curve by tucking in your chin, then pulling in your navel to the spine to control your torso and maintain a taut stomach.

67

Abdominal and back strength

The exercises on pages 68–69 condition the deep-seated muscles that support your back, enhancing your core stability.

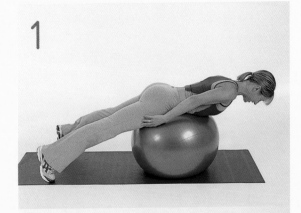

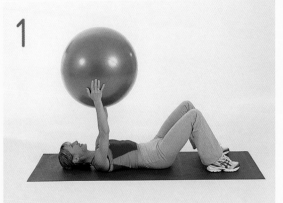

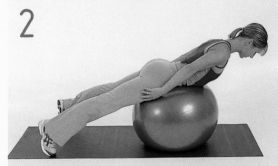

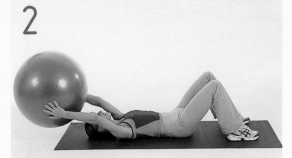

Human cannonball

Strengthens your lower back and buttock muscles. Work on a non-slip surface or brace your feet against a wall.

1 Lie with your stomach and hips on the ball, and chest, head and neck off it. Keep your neck long and shoulders relaxed. Place your hands at your sides. Keep your legs apart and press into your feet for support.

2 Keeping your chin tucked in, raise your body slightly and then lower back to the start position.

Ab-alert

Increases awareness of the muscles that form a major part of your core strength. Work slowly for maximum benefit.

1 Lie on your back with your knees bent and feet hip-width apart. Place hands on each side of the ball and hold it up at chest level, with elbows slightly bent. Pull your navel in towards the spine and straighten your arms to lift the ball upwards.

2 Slowly move the ball behind your head. You will feel your spine arching off the floor. Pull in your navel even more and narrow the gap between your ribs and hips. Return the ball to the start position.

1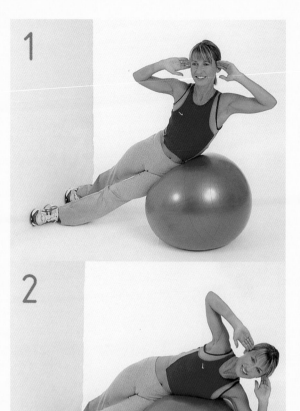

2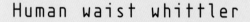

1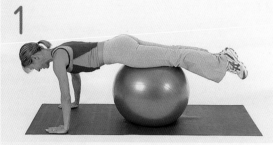

2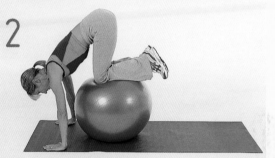

3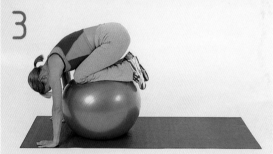

Human waist whittler

Targets the oblique muscles at the sides of your waist and works stomach and back muscles to maintain balance and control. Keep your head in line with your spine to avoid pulling on your neck.

1 Brace your feet in a stride position against a step or wall. With the ball under the side of your body at hip level, pull in your navel and place your fingertips on your temples. Keep your elbows back and squeeze your shoulder blades together.

2 Slowly lower and arch your body sideways over the ball. Keep your abdominal muscles firmly contracted as you slowly rise to the start position.

Knees up

Strengthens your stomach and arms, working several muscle groups together. Keep your navel pulled in towards your spine to stabilize your back.

1 Start with your thighs on the ball, your navel pulled in and your shoulders over your hands.

2 Bend your legs and draw your knees inwards. Keep your arms stable.

3 Continue drawing your knees up towards your chest, until you reach the position shown. Return to the start position, using your stomach muscles to maintain control.

Leg strength

The exercises on pages 70–71 are designed to work on the different muscles in your legs.

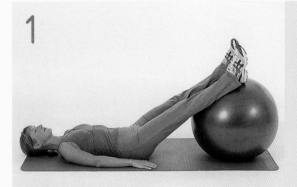

Ball drag

Targets your buttocks, backs of legs, calves, lower back, pelvic floor and core stabilizing muscles.

1 Lie on the floor with your legs straight and heels and calves resting on the ball. Place your arms at your sides, your palms face down, and relax your neck and shoulders.

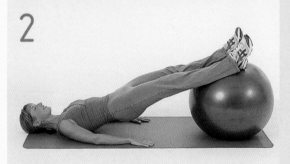

2 Tighten your buttocks, pull your navel in towards the spine and lift your hips upwards until your legs and shoulders form a diagonal line. Press down into your feet to avoid your back arching.

3 Push down into the ball through your feet and pull the ball in towards your buttocks as far as you can. Keep the buttocks lifted. You will feel the muscles working from the calves through to the buttocks.

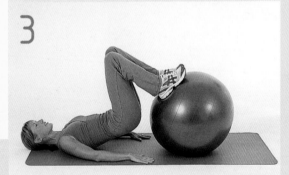

4 Push into the ball and slowly straighten your legs out again, keeping the ball steady. Lower your hips back to the start position.

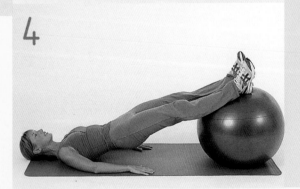

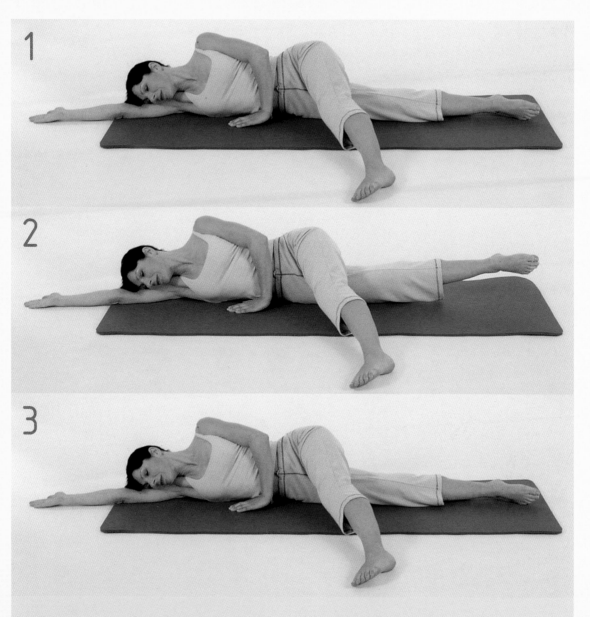

1

2

3

Inner thigh lift

1 Lie on your side with your ear, middle of shoulder, hip and ankle all in a straight line and feet pointing down. Place the upper arm on the floor in front of you; stretch the lower arm out above your head, palm up, with your head resting on the arm. Bring your upper leg in front of you so that the foot of your upper leg rests on the floor, keeping the leg straight and one hip stacked on top of the other.

2 Exhale, drawing in the abdominals, and stretch your lower leg away from you as you slowly lift the heel about 15 cm (6 in) off the mat. Make sure you keep your lower knee facing forwards throughout and that your hips don't move.

3 Inhale as you lower your leg to the mat. Repeat 6–10 times each side.

Advanced balance and stability

This is a more challenging Pilates exercise, requiring greater abdominal, back and leg strength. Don't perform this exercise if you have a back injury.

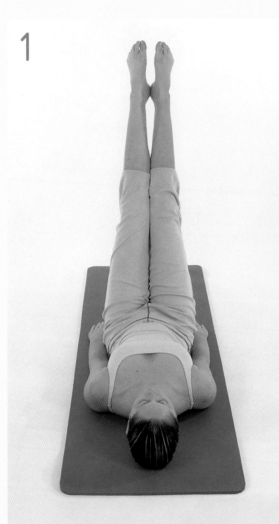

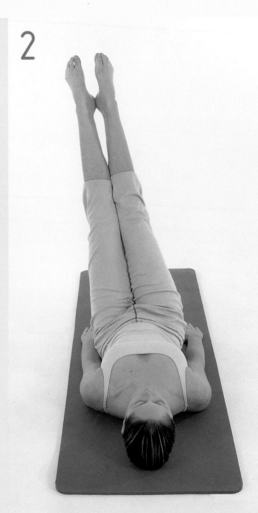

Corkscrew

1 Lie on your back with your arms by your sides. Press your palms into the mat for extra stability. Lift and straighten your legs up to the ceiling at a 90 degree angle to the mat. Turn your legs out, engaging your lower buttock muscles throughout. Your inner thighs will also engage.

2 Inhale and take your legs over to one side without allowing your body to lift.

3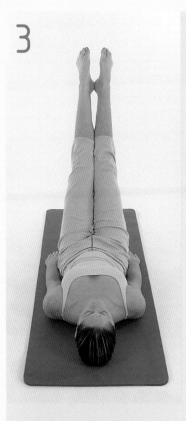

4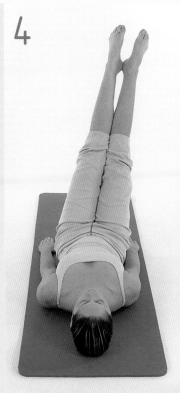

5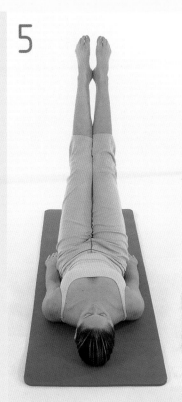

3 Exhale, drawing in your abdominals, as you circle your legs down through the centre line of your body.

4 Continue exhaling as you continue the circle over to the other side.

5 Continue exhaling as you circle the knees back up and in to the centre. To reverse the movement, inhale and take your legs over to the other side. Then exhale, drawing in the abdominals, and circle your legs down, around and back to the centre. Repeat 5 circles each side, alternating the direction.

Top training tip

The key to Pilates is the breathing, and this takes practice. You need to learn to breathe from underneath your ribcage, on top of your pelvis (pubic bone area). Open your chest and stand relaxed. The breathing is lateral thoracic breathing, which means movement should be expanding out towards your lower back, in a very controlled and slow manner.

A running strategy for beginners

In the initial stages of your running programme, you should be looking to walk or walk-run three times a week with days of rest in between – on Sunday, Tuesday and Thursday or Friday, for example. As you progress, you will be able to walk, walk-run or run four to five days a week. But remember the principles of training. Don't increase everything at the same time – you can run for longer, run faster or run more often, but not all in the same week (see 'Key principles of training', pages 46–47).

Once you are more confident in your running, you will be able to work your way along the continuum below until you can run for 10, 20, 40, 60 minutes and beyond, across a variety of terrains, using different running methods and a range of pacing. The continuum does not need to be followed in any particular order, although for a beginner it makes sense to progress through the stages of running as you get fitter and stronger.

WALK ➤ POWER WALK ➤ WALK-RUN ➤ EASY RUN ➤ STEADY RUN ➤ TEMPO RUN ➤ LONG RUN ➤ FARTLEK ➤ INTERVALS ➤ HILLS ➤ SPEED WORK

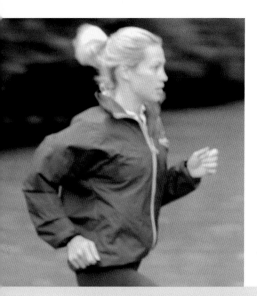

This schedule is to get you running competently for 30 minutes within 30 days of training. The days on which you run don't have to be consecutive – you can adapt them to fit in with your schedule. For example, Day 1 might be a Sunday, Day 2 a Wednesday and Day 3 a Friday. Take as much time as you need to progress; everyone is different and you might achieve the 30 minute run in fewer, or more, than 30 days. Feel free to repeat any of the days or to step back a couple of days and move forwards again when ready. Try walking one day, resting the next. It is okay to walk on consecutive days, but make sure you take regular days off.

An easy walk is a casual stroll. A steady walk means picking up your speed, with noticeable changes in your breathing rate; a pace at which you can still talk, but need to concentrate to maintain. Brisk walking is power walking (see page 60). Instructions in brackets indicate intervals (see page 63).

30 days to 30 minutes schedule

Beginners are unlikely to be able to start a running programme with actual running. Instead, you will begin with walking and build up the frequency, intensity and duration of exercise until regular, steady running is possible. The rate at which you achieve this will depend on a variety of factors including your history of exercise participation, present fitness level, body shape, weight, genes, diet and the amount of time and effort you invest in the initial walking-running programme.

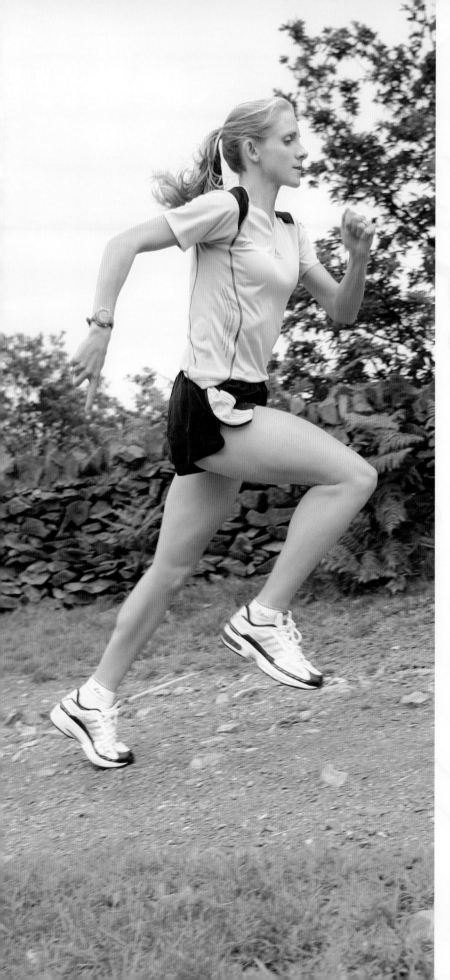

Top training tip

Keeping a diary of your physical activity is a great way of monitoring your progress. It is especially useful if you are preparing for a specific event, as you can look back through your notes to establish your patterns of training and see when real improvements were made, when you felt tired and when you ran well. A training diary should include how long you ran for (in time or distance), where you ran, what the weather was like, the type of running that you did and how you felt.

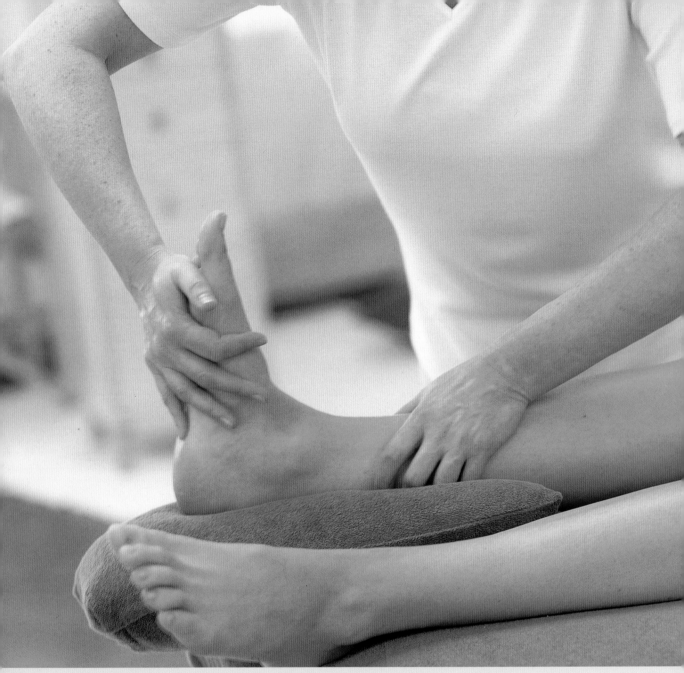

When not to run

Nobody feels 100 per cent all year round and there will be the odd occasion when you question whether it is a good idea to go out and run or not. Perhaps you have incurred an injury, are battling with a nasty cold or simply feel under the weather. The following pages outline the physical hurdles you may encounter as a woman runner and offer advice on how to deal with them.

Common running injuries

The key to dealing with injuries is really prevention – that is, taking the appropriate action to avoid getting injured in the first place. This means listening closely to your body and seeking professional advice as soon as anything feels tight or sore beyond normal levels. Ignoring these niggles is likely to lead to them getting worse. This does not mean you have to stop running, but it is important to seek advice so that you can counteract any problems straight away. This chapter describes the most common problems, along with ways of avoiding them.

Knee pain and iliotibial band (ITB) syndrome

Women runners can be susceptible to knee problems due to the angle of the thigh bone in relation to the wider female pelvis. This causes the kneecap to pull away from the midline during weight-bearing activities, particularly when a woman is standing on one leg – as is the case when running. Knee or iliotibial band pain can be accentuated by any deficiency in the buttock muscle called the gluteus medius, which lifts the thigh outwards from the hip.

Advice: Shoes that have motion control may reduce or prevent the tendency of the kneecap to slide outside its normal course. A prescription orthotic may also help (see 'The right footwear', pages 24–25).

Developing strength in the gluteus medius can also help, as this will create a more stable alignment for the kneecap and put less strain on the iliotibial band. Regular stretching of the iliotibial band will also help. To prevent imbalances occurring, it is a good idea to follow a muscle-strengthening programme that takes in all muscle groups. Quadricep-muscle strengthening on the leg-extension machine in the gym is often beneficial for general knee pain, but can be counterproductive if it is not done in conjunction with strengthening of the flexors, abductors and adductors in the thigh. Seek advice at your local gym.

Sports massage

Having your legs massaged by a qualified sports therapist or masseur is a wonderful treat for tired runners. It is relaxing, flushes out the muscles, promotes circulation and can help ward off potential injury. Go on, try it!

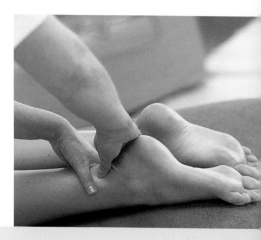

Liz says: 'Before you start any regular exercise programme, it's a good idea to have a medical check-up with your doctor.'

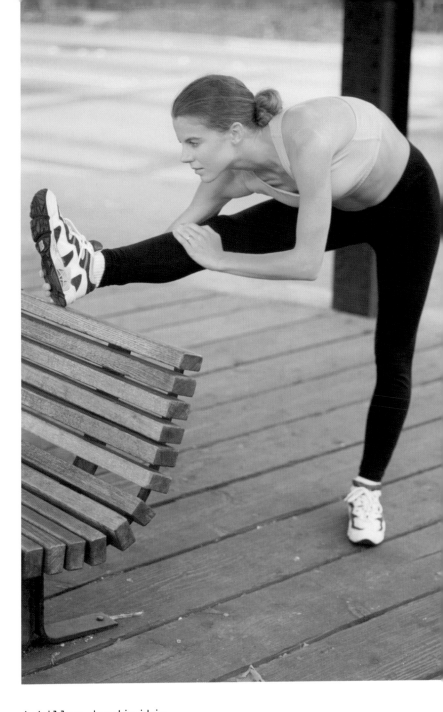

Achilles tendinitis

High-heeled shoes put pressure on the ball of the foot and can cause pain in the metatarsals and nerves at the front of the foot. They also shorten the Achilles tendon by tightening the calf, which can lead to a typical overuse injury such as chronic Achilles tendinitis or a heel spur.

Advice: Warm up well, with plenty of stretching after running, holding each stretch for 20–30 seconds. Try facing a wall with your hands against it and leaning forwards with a straight body, keeping both heels on the ground until you feel your calf muscles and Achilles tendon stretch. Standing with the ball of the foot on a solid step and allowing the heel to drop is also useful. Ease the stretch further every ten seconds if you can.

Foot and toe deformities

If a woman has a flat foot or pronates excessively (see page 25), or has weak or unstable ankle ligaments, she has a greater chance of developing foot and toe problems such as bunions. The problem is often compounded by shoes designed primarily for the male foot (the female forefoot is wider and the hind foot narrower).

Advice: Wear women's running shoes designed for motion control and stability. If necessary, see a sports doctor to get a prescription orthotic to control the excessive pronation. Ankle-strengthening exercises and off-road running over uneven surfaces will strengthen ligaments and stabilize the ankle.

Scoliosis

This curvature of the spine is most prevalent in female adolescents. In runners, it can contribute to lower back and hip pain. It can also cause a pelvic tilt, where one limb acts 'longer' than the other. This almost always develops into an overuse injury to the 'shorter' limb.

Advice: See a podiatrist who can equalize limb length either through a prescription orthotic or a heel lift. This treatment will reduce the potential for overuse injuries.

Stress fractures

These result from biomechanical stress on a weakened bone. If you are a heavier runner, have very poor technique or do long distances, you are more at risk. The prevalence of such an injury increases dramatically as weekly distances exceed 32 km (20 miles). A decrease in bone-mineral density owing to osteoporosis or poor nutrition through eating disorders can contribute.

Advice: Make sure you have the right shoes for your weight, distance and running style. Demineralization of the bone requires medical attention, a proper diet and psychological help if the cause is an eating disorder. Complete rest from running is necessary to allow for complete healing.

Blisters

When two surfaces – such as skin and sock – rub together, friction is generated and blisters can develop. A blister is a fluid-filled pocket that lies beneath the surface of the skin. Fortunately, there are steps you can take to keep blisters away.

- Choose the right shoes (see pages 24–25). They should fit comfortably: too narrow, and they cause blisters on the big and little toes; too loose, and they cause blisters on the tips of the toes.
- Decrease the potential for friction by wearing good-quality running socks that carry moisture away from the skin.
- Try adding talcum powder to the inside of your socks to dry your feet, or petroleum jelly to reduce rubbing.
- Apply specialist blister protection pads. Make sure they are thin and don't generate rubbing in other places.

Safety first

Listen to your body. The more you run, the more proficient you will become at interpreting your sensations. If you feel sudden sharp pains in your chest, stop immediately and book an appointment with your doctor. Refer to a qualified sports physiotherapist if you have sudden, painful twinges or spasms in your muscles that don't go away with a few minutes' walking, or the onset of persistent joint pain.

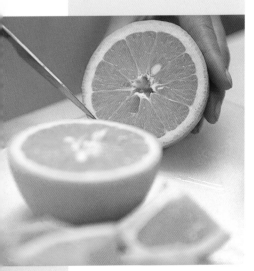

Dealing with a blister

Blisters can be painful, but usually clear up with a little gentle persuasion:
- Clean the area with antiseptic soap.
- Drain the blister by puncturing the edge using a sterile needle.
- Gently squeeze to remove the fluid.
- Leave the roof of the blister attached.
- Apply antibacterial solution.
- Ensure that the area is kept clean and dry.
- Attach a specialist blister 'second skin' plaster to promote healing.
- Keep the dressing fresh and watch for any infection.

Colds, coughs and common complaints

There will be times when you feel under the weather; the key is knowing when to rest. It is possible to run with a light head cold, but keep it slow and wrap up warm. Don't run if your symptoms are accompanied by a sore throat, swollen glands, a chesty cough, aching muscles and dizziness or fever. Seek medical advice and avoid running until all your symptoms have cleared. Minor coughs and colds usually clear up on their own within a week or two and you will be able to slowly ease yourself back into your normal running routine. Don't get back into it too quickly or you could invite your illness to return.

Menstruation

There is no reason not to run when you are menstruating. By balancing some of the hormonal fluctuations, running can be great at reducing the symptoms associated with premenstrual tension (PMT), such as breast tenderness, bloating and general fatigue. If you know what to expect, it will be easier to continue with your normal running schedule. It may help to keep a note in your training diary about how you feel each day. You may notice a pattern of fatigue or of feeling more energized on specific days associated with your monthly cycle.

Running and pregnancy

It is a good idea to stay physically active during pregnancy and that can certainly include running. Continue with familiar exercise, adjusting the level of your activity as your pregnancy progresses. Try to stand tall when you exercise: keeping an upright posture while you run will help to work the deep abdominals as they lengthen and soften during pregnancy.

First trimester

You may have concerns about the effects of exercising during the very early stages, especially if this is your first child, but it is possible to continue as normal. Consider wearing a heart-rate monitor to make sure you don't work too hard (see page 26), and watch the terrain – keep off rough, undulating ground to limit the risk of falling.

As your size increases, you may experience shortness of breath, which can be attributed to the increased demands placed by pregnancy on the cardiovascular system. At this time, you may feel heavy and less light on your feet, and raging hormones, sore breasts and lethargy may sometimes mean you might want to consider cycling and gym work instead. Pelvic or lower back pain may occur if the joint and ligament softening that begins to occur early in pregnancy is not well controlled by the stabilizing muscles of the pelvis. If that is the case, reduce impact exercise and seek professional advice.

Second and third trimesters

Energy levels could return in the second trimester, as morning sickness decreases, and it should still be possible to run, with cycling and swimming as alternative activities. If you continue to run, make sure someone always knows when and where you are training and try to have your partner or a friend accompany you. By the third trimester, it is sensible to exercise at the gym.

Stress incontinence is a slight leaking of urine associated with an increase in activity, such as laughing, coughing, sneezing or running, and is very common in the later stages of pregnancy. It is fine to continue exercising, but you may want to wear some protection, such as a panty liner.

Running post-birth

Finding the appropriate time to return to taking exercise and especially running will vary for every mother. It is important to get the medical all clear to resume training, to listen to your body and to take into consideration your new circumstances. It is unlikely that you will be able to slide right back into your old running routine, and you will need to allow time to develop a new one.

It is now widely accepted that normal levels of exercise will not adversely affect the volume or composition of breast milk. For your comfort, it is probably best to exercise after feeding and to wear a well-fitting and supportive bra. Make sure you adequately replenish your fluids and calories post-exercise, ready for the next feed.

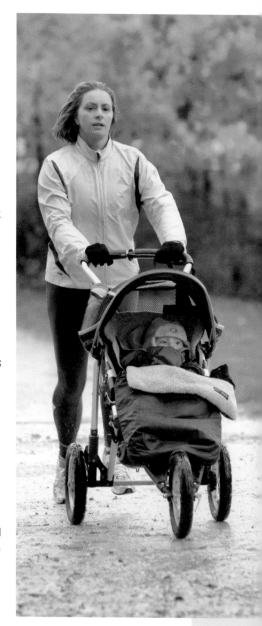

.GO!...READY...

STEADY...GO!..

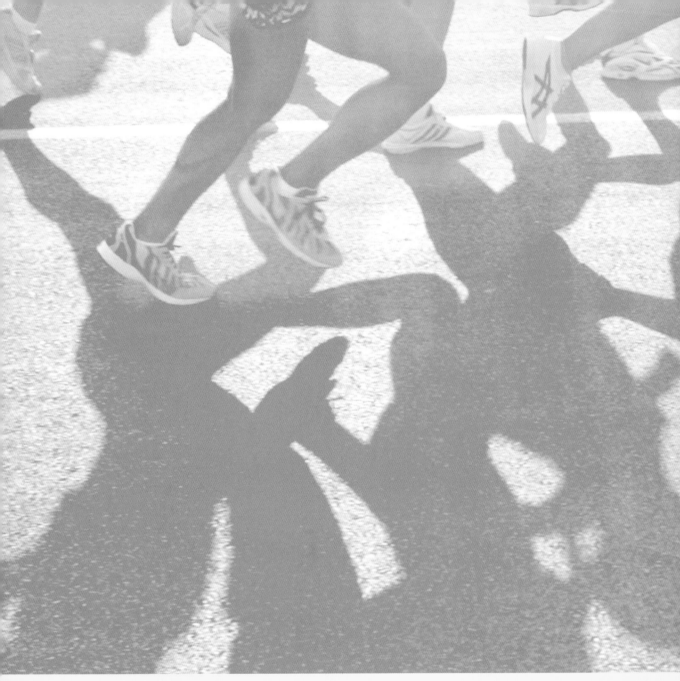

Let's go

By now you will have completed the 30 days to 30 minutes schedule (see page 79) and will be able to run non-stop for half an hour. You may also have tackled the first 10 week training schedule (see pages 81–82). At the very least, you will have started running and will be trying different types of running training, you will have taken on board the key principles of training and will be building up your workout sessions progressively.

Encouraging you to take your running one step further, this last section of the book guides you through all there is to know about participating in a running event. With so many different options open to you, it can be difficult to know where to start, so you'll find an outline of each major type of running event, including road running, cross county, mixed sex and women only, to help you decide which ones are for you.

There is advice on how to choose and enter an event, as well as guidance on getting ready to race. Find out how to prepare for an event, what to do the day before and on the day itself, and pick up some tips for running a better race. Your performance will improve significantly if you approach the big day well prepared, relaxed, confident and ready to perform.

Motivation is crucial when you are running longer distances or training for a specific event. This section suggests ways of boosting your morale and commitment, by setting realistic short- and long-term goals and perhaps joining a running group or hiring a training coach for extra support.

Most importantly, this final section of the book also provides 10 week and 12 week training schedules that will enable you to prepare for specific events – 5 km (3.1 miles), 10 km (6.2 miles), half-marathon and marathon. For each distance, the schedules cater for a range of abilities, from beginner to improver to competent. Select an appropriate schedule for your ability and desired event, progressing to the next level when you need more of a challenge. Following a schedule is at the heart of good race preparation; it will add variety and structure to your running and keep you focused and motivated.

Liz says: 'Congratulations on getting this far! Now you're ready to start training for real events.'

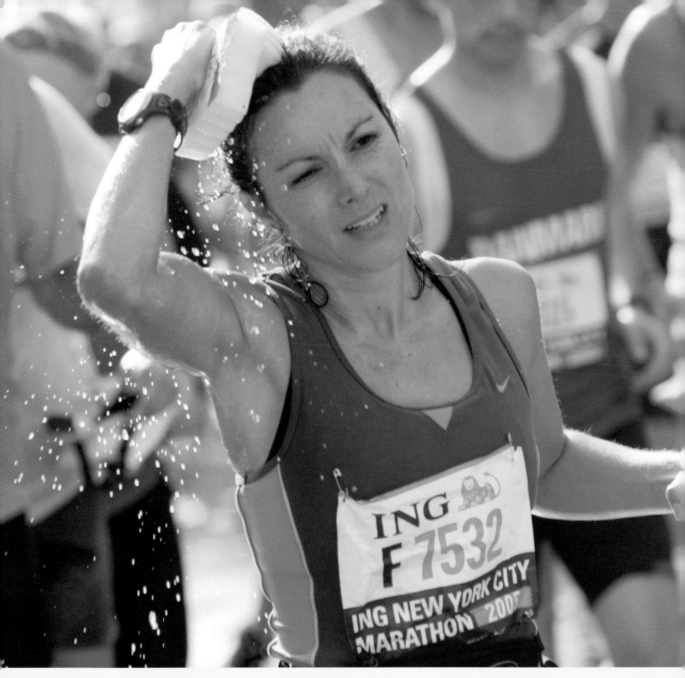

Running events

It can be daunting even to consider running a race. The key is to think of it as an 'event' – you don't have to 'race', although you might like to try to set a personal best. If you have that intrinsic competitive streak, you will relish the challenge a race offers, but rest assured that competition is not compulsory.

Types of event

- **Road running:** This is the most common and usually the most accessible type of event, staged just about everywhere and ranging from small-scale local events (50–100 runners) to mass-participation city events (40,000 runners or more). Distances vary, but are usually fixed at some common distances: 5 km (3.1 miles), 10 km (6.2 miles), half-marathon (21 km/13.1 miles) and marathon (42 km/26.2 miles). Mass-participation events are often oversubscribed and to get in you have to enter very early or through a lottery system, or by raising money for charity. Such events are a brilliant way to get a real challenge and adventure from your running. The vast majority of road-running events are on a smaller scale, however, and much more accessible. You can almost guarantee there will be one in your home town or city.
- **Cross-country events:** These are organized running races that take you off road and into the country. Usually, they are set up through running clubs, districts or regions, but there are also open events. Expect to get wet and muddy but have lots of fun at the same time. (See also the information about multi-terrain and trail races, below.)
- **Track racing:** A running track is a 400 m (¼ mile) oval made of rubber tartan. Track races for runners are usually, but not always, reserved for club runners, although there are some open events for anyone to enter. They are always timed and run over set distances.
- **Multi-terrain and trail races:** These are running events that follow footpaths, trails and routes in the countryside. They often cover approximate distances and really allow you to enjoy the fresh air and the whole off-road racing experience.
- **Walk-runs:** Some events are billed exclusively as walk-run events, where it is expected that everyone will walk and jog a little.
- **Fell/hill running:** Races that take place up and down mountains.
- **Ultra-distance races:** Long events that usually take place over around 80 km (50 miles), and demand a great deal of preparation.

Women-only events

Most road-running races see men and women running together, but women-only races are growing in popularity. Their advantages include:

- *The realization that other women, just like you, participate in running events.*
- *An opportunity to raise money for women-focused charities.*
- *Encouraging women to enjoy being active.*
- *A chance to participate in a less intimidating setting.*
- *Less pressure to perform, but the opportunity to reach personal goals.*
- *Having fun, meeting new friends and enjoying the company of fellow women.*

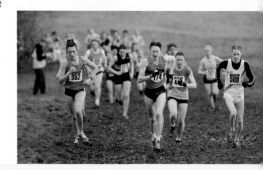

Confidence booster

There will always be other runners of your standard. People of all shapes, sizes, abilities, backgrounds, nationalities – able and disabled – participate in running events, which are simply communities of friendly people drawn together by their love of running.

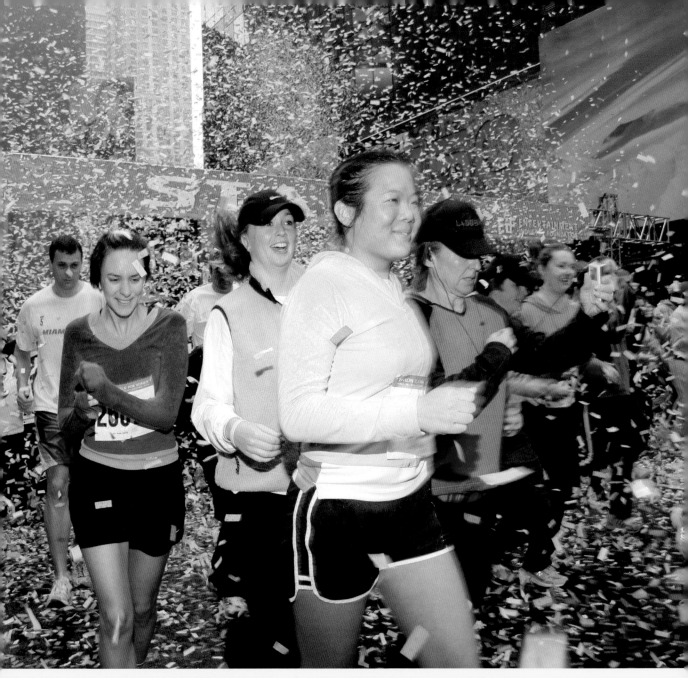

Choosing a running event

There are literally thousands of running events to choose from. In order to find one that suits you, you need to consider a number of important questions. What type of event appeals to you? How far would you like to run? What is your current state of running fitness? How long do you have to prepare for the event? How far can you travel? How much will it cost to enter?

A race for everyone

Road-running events are the most common events and the most accessible, especially to first-timers. Choose one that is appropriate to your experience and fitness. Don't expect to run a marathon as your first race, with hardly any experience and little or no time to prepare. It is a good idea to look for a small local event, where you will not have far to travel, no pre-event accommodation to worry about and you may know the route and other participants. Finding an event that attracts a large number of runners is also a good idea. The bigger the field, the more likely that there will be other women runners of your standard. You will get a real buzz from being with other runners. Big races also attract big crowds, so there will be plenty of support. And don't worry: not everyone will be better, faster or more professional than you.

Where to look

Specialist running magazines are a good place to start looking for an event. They contain race listings or race diaries that typically show all the events taking place over the forthcoming months. They usually give details of date, distance, race headquarters/venue, start time, cost, where to send entries, number of entries in previous years and terrain. Online running websites usually contain extensive race listings, and many individual events have their own websites. Other women runners are also an invaluable source of information, offering their personal experiences of running events.

How to enter

Once you have chosen a race, it is a good idea to enter in advance. For the majority of races, you can enter a few months, a few weeks or a few days before, or even on the day of the event. Enter with plenty of time to prepare: at least a month for a shorter race and much longer for a marathon. Many mass-participation races are notoriously difficult to get into and you have to enter a long time in advance, in some cases up to 12 months.

Top training tip

Points to consider when choosing an event:
- *Your motives for entering*
- *Type of event*
- *Location*
- *Terrain*
- *Distance*
- *How long you have for training*
- *Closing date for entries*
- *Start time*
- *Entry cost*
- *Standard – race listings often show the last finisher's time*
- *What you get for participating – some races offer medals, T-shirts and so on*

Liz says: 'Choose a race and get your entry in. Entering in advance will give you a target to aim for and a real focus in your training.'

Taking the panic out of race day

- **Before the day:** Enter and pay in advance. You will be sent a race number or told how to collect it on the day. If the race is early in the morning and far from home, consider booking accommodation for the night before.
- **One day to go:** Pack your kit bag. Don't forget to include your race number and some safety pins to attach it to your vest or T-shirt. Take spare clean clothes and shoes to wear after the race and a post-race snack. Make sure you have read any race-day information. Find out about the course/route and where to park your car, and double check the start time.
- **The big day:** Eat a light breakfast – some cereal, a bagel or some toast two to three hours before the event usually works best, kick-starting your metabolism and supplying your body with energy. Drink water, juice or an energy drink in the hours before the event.

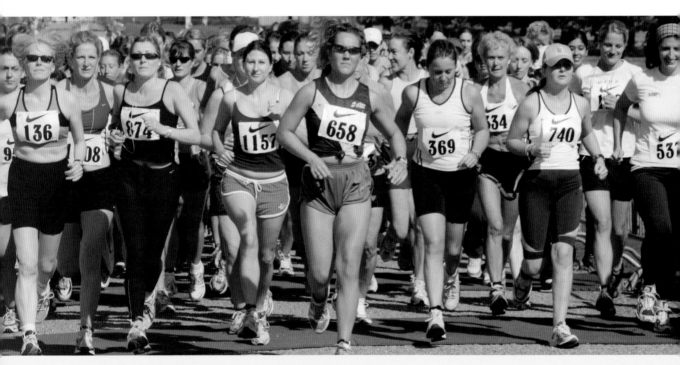

Getting ready to race

Worried about what to wear, what you need to take, whether you will get lost and what to do at the start and finish? The key to a successful and enjoyable race day lies in the planning and preparation. Your training programme should have taken care of your running fitness, so relax and enjoy the experience of participating in an event.

Finding your level

Whether you are preparing for a 5 km (3.1 mile), 10 km (6.2 mile), half-marathon (21 km/13.1 mile) or marathon (42 km/26.2 mile) event, in each case you will find a schedule designed for beginner, improver and competent runners. Evaluate your performance before choosing a category. Remember that before starting on any of these running schedules you should have completed, or be able to complete, the 30 days to 30 minutes running schedule (see page 79).

- **Beginner:** You are a beginner if you have very little experience of running and are relatively new to exercise. You should start your training very gently and slowly. You will have completed the 30 days to 30 minutes schedule, but you may now be nervous about how to proceed and a little uncertain of what to expect. You aim to do two or three workouts in your regular week. You may have no real idea as to what sort of speed you run at and may not be convinced that you will enter an event, but you are enthusiastic and ready to go.

- **Improver:** If you are an improver, you have a little experience of running and are physically active on a regular basis. You will be able to run without stopping for 30 minutes or more. You will be a little more confident in your ability than a beginner and you know what it feels like to run at different speeds. You aim to run three or four times a week. You might have entered and completed a few races of varying distances and even have personal bests for these.

- **Competent:** If you are at competent level, you are an experienced regular runner who can run non-stop for an hour or longer. You are familiar with different types of running training, such as fartlek, intervals and tempo runs, and have some racing experience at a variety of distances. You know what your weekly distance levels and running speeds are. You aim to run three to six times a week. You consider yourself to have reached a good level of running fitness, and are looking to develop your running, improve your personal bests and run faster.

Key to schedules

- *Easy walk = strolling*
- *Steady walk = picking up some speed*
- *Brisk walk = power walking (see page 60)*
- *Easy run = very light jogging*
- *Steady run = running with more effort, breathing harder*
- *Hard run = faster running, with concentration*
- *Fartlek = varied pace running*
- *Intervals = repetition of hard running with recovery periods (instructions in brackets)*
- *Tempo = running on the threshold of comfort*

Liz says: 'Think, feel and act like a runner, and you *are* a runner!'

Tapering:

- *Before an event, you should taper your training, reducing volume and intensity. Never complete the hardest run of the week the day or even two or three days before an event.*
- *The longer the race, the greater the tapering process. For example, a marathon taper may begin three weeks before the race, with mileage decreasing by 30 per cent each week.*
- *For a 5 km (3.1 mile) event, you might do a sharper, speedier run on the Monday or Tuesday of race week, followed by gentle running on other days.*

Adapting the schedules

You can tweak these schedules to fit your own lifestyle and commitments. As long as the type of running stays the same, there's no reason why you can't run on different days of the week. For example, instead of running on a Monday, Tuesday, Thursday and Saturday, you might run on Monday, Wednesday, Friday and Sunday. Remember the key principles of training, however (see pages 46–47). Your plan must be progressive, should include different types of running at different speeds and should always include rest and recovery. Don't do all your running at the weekend. On active recovery days, either rest or go to the gym, go for a light swim or go for a walk. You can also move up or down a category if you find your current programme either too easy or too demanding.

Boost your training

- **Rest:** As a rule of thumb, for every hard day take two days easy.
- **Plan:** Keep a training diary to record your week's training and goals, in order to check progress and keep yourself on track.
- **Vary your pace:** After an initial settling period of three to six weeks, you should start varying the pace of your runs. This will keep you interested and make sure you carry on improving. If you are training for a specific race, train at and above the pace you are hoping to run. Know your 1.6 km (1 mile) race time splits (see the pace chart on page 101) and pace your training appropriately.
- **Vary your running route:** This will stop you getting in a rut. Run your normal course in reverse or go exploring.
- **Ease the pressure:** Try going for a run for duration (for 20 minutes, for example), rather than running a set distance.
- **Establish a routine:** Make getting out there as simple as possible by establishing a regular routine. Running at a certain time on a certain day will soon become second nature.
- **Get some support:** Find a training partner or running advisor. You can get specific guidance about your running from a qualified running coach or specialist (see page 105).
- **Get the right kit:** Make sure you wear breathable running clothing (see pages 22–24). Maintaining the correct body temperature will help to make your runs easier and more successful.
- **Fuel up:** Keep the basic healthy eating principles in mind. Eat sensibly and in moderation from all food groups (see 'What to eat', pages 28–33).
- **Race:** Racing provides a great target to aim for and will help you to settle into a routine, run regularly, lose weight, tone up and achieve everything else running offers.

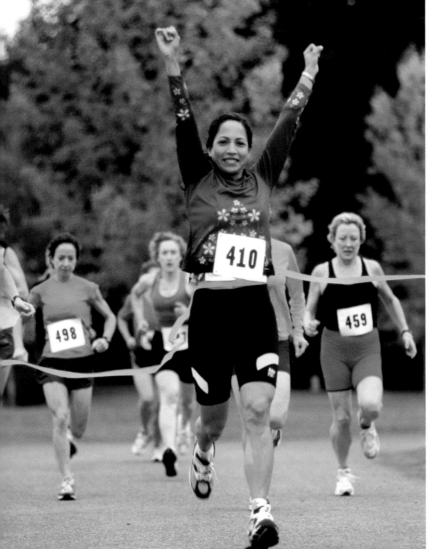

Your first races

- Get to know the course before the race.
- Pace judgement is crucial: don't start too fast and concentrate on maintaining your race pace.
- Stay focused on your own progress and motivated by your goals.
- If you are in a mixed race, use the men to 'hide' and pull away from your female competitors.
- If it is windy, conserve your energy by taking shelter behind runners going at a similar pace to you.
- Harness your mental potential. Use visualization beforehand, picturing yourself running the way you want to run, and continue to think positively during the race.
- Know that it is going to feel hard and uncomfortable. Be driven.
- Always go for a sprint at the finish.

Running 5 km (3.1 miles) and 10 km (6.2 miles)

Before you begin training for your 5 km (3.1 mile) or 10 km (6.2 mile) event, consider what you hope to achieve. Your goal might be to run the entire event without stopping, or simply to finish the event. You may want the personal challenge of running faster than you have before, or of beating a fellow competitor. Whatever your goal, remember that by far the most important strategy in any racing is the training – get that right and you will run well.

	WEEK 1	WEEK 2	WEEK 3	WEEK 4	WEEK 5
MON	Active recovery.	Active recovery.	Active recovery.	Active recovery.	Active recovery.
TUES	15 min easy walk-run.	2 min brisk walk, 5 min easy run, 2 min brisk walk, 5 min easy run, 2 min brisk walk, 3 min easy run.	3 min easy run, (3 min hard run, 2 min easy walk. Repeat x3).	3 min easy run, (2 min hard run, 5 min easy run. Repeat x3).	20 min easy run.
WED	Rest.	Rest.	Rest.	Rest.	Rest.
THURS	(2 min brisk walk, 2 min easy run, 1 min steady walk, 3 min easy run. Repeat x2.)	2 min easy run, 10 min steady run, 5 min brisk walk.	5 min easy run, 10 min steady run, 5 min easy run.	5 min easy run, 15 min steady run, 5 min easy run.	35 min easy run.
FRI	Rest.	Rest.	Rest.	Rest.	Rest.
SAT/ SUN	3 min steady walk, 15 min easy run, 5 min steady walk.	3 min brisk walk, 20 min easy run, 3 min steady walk.	2 min brisk walk, 30 min easy run, 2 min brisk walk.	35 min easy run.	45 min easy run.

5 km (3.1 miles): Beginner 10 week schedule

In Weeks 1–5 start and finish with a 3 minute easy walk. End your workout with stretching exercises. Monday is an active recovery day – go to the gym or for a swim. Tuesday is for adding pace. Wednesday, Friday and Saturday or Sunday are rest days. Thursday is for speed. Your weekend running day is for building endurance.

	WEEK 7	WEEK 8	WEEK 9	WEEK 10	WEEK 11	WEEK 12
MON	30 min steady run.	45 min easy run.	30 min easy run.	30 min steady run.	Rest.	Rest.
TUES	10 min easy run, (3 min hard run, 3 min easy run. Repeat x5), 10 min easy run.	10 min easy run, (4 min hard run, 2 min easy run. Repeat x5), 10 min easy run.	10 min easy run, (5 min hard run, 90 sec easy run. Repeat x4), 10 min easy run.	10 min easy run, (6 min hard run, 2 min easy run. Repeat x4), 10 min easy run.	10 min easy run, (1 min hard run, 1 min very easy run. Repeat x5), 5 min easy run.	5 min easy run, (1 min hard run, 1 min walk. Repeat x3), 5 min easy run.
WED	Active recovery.	Active recovery.	Active recovery.	Active recovery.	Active recovery.	Active recovery.
THURS	45 min steady run.	50 min steady run.	60 min easy run.	45 min easy run.	25 min easy run.	Rest.
FRI	Rest.	Rest.	Rest.	Rest.	Rest.	Rest.
SAT	5 min easy run, 20 min hard run, 5 min easy run.	5 min easy run, 30 min tempo run, 10 min easy run.	20 min easy run, 10 min hard run, 10 min easy run.	5 min easy run, 30 min fartlek, 5 min easy run.	10 min easy run, 25 min tempo, 10 min easy run.	10 min easy run.
SUN	85 min easy run.	90 min easy run.	80 min steady run.	75 min easy run.	60 min easy run.	RACE DAY

Liz says: 'Avoid comparing yourself to others. Remember how far *you* have come and how much *you* have achieved.'

Top training tips

Race hydration:
- *A supply of fluids is essential when you run long distances, to rehydrate you and replace energy stores. Commercial sports energy drinks are a good option, providing a blend of fluids and nutrients (see page 35).*
- *During a long run, aim to drink at 20 minute intervals. Sip a little at a time and take three to five sips each time.*
- *Fluids can be carried with a fuel belt or camelback (see page 27).*
- *An energy drink in a sports bottle could be placed at a convenient point on a loop course, for you to pick up during the run.*
- *If you are training, an enthusiastic helper could ride a bike next to you and pass you a drinks bottle at the appropriate stages in your run.*

Half-marathon training strategy

- Be flexible but sensible with your running schedules. Don't attempt too much too quickly, but build up strength, stamina and skill gradually.
- Don't be afraid to take a day's rest if you become tired, but allow the schedule to test you when appropriate.
- Ensure that your running is progressive: include a variety of training types in your schedule (see pages 60–63).
- Always warm up and cool down properly to avoid injury (see pages 52–59).
- Join a running group (see page 105) or find a running buddy.
- Keep a training diary.

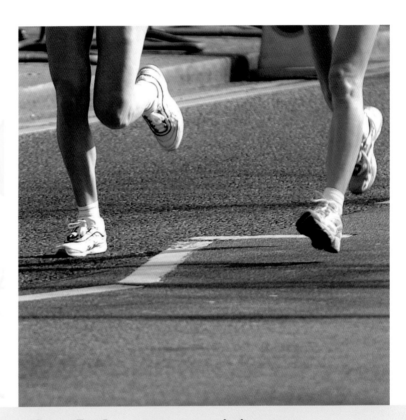

Running a half-marathon

If you have decided to run a half-marathon or a marathon, select your training schedules carefully. Your preparation for a challenging event like this should be progressive, steadily building up to the longer distances. If you are a total beginner, start with the 30 days to 30 minutes schedule (see page 79), then progress to one of the easier 5 km (3.1 mile) or 10 km (6.2 mile) schedules. Only once you have completed a higher level 5 km (3.1 mile) or a 10 km (6.2 mile) schedule will you be ready for half-marathon or marathon training.

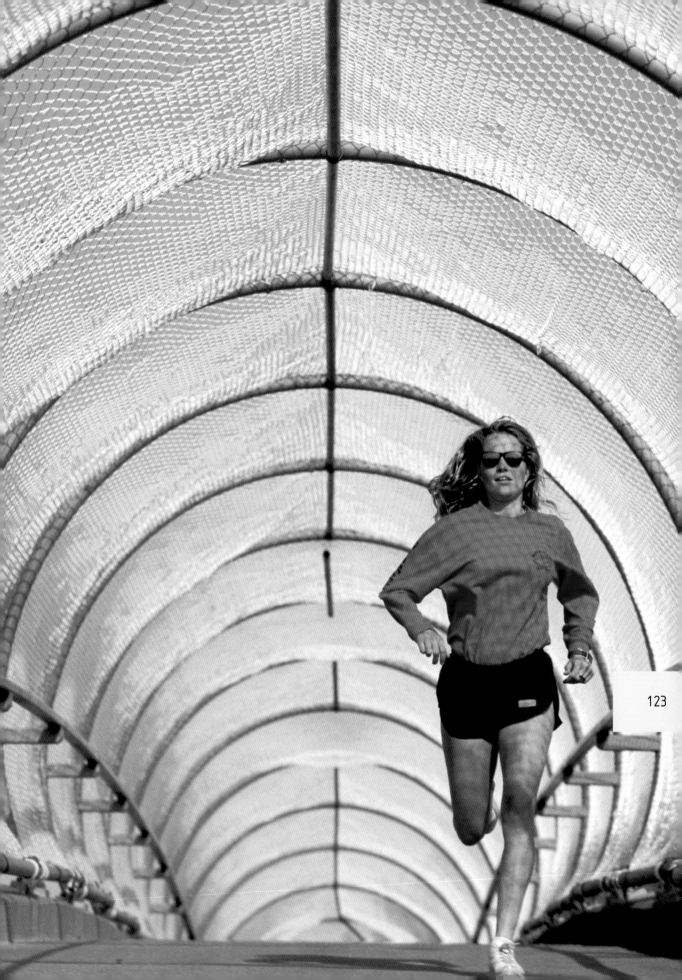

	WEEK 1	WEEK 2	WEEK 3	WEEK 4	WEEK 5	WEEK 6
MON	Rest/active recovery.	Rest/active recovery.	Rest/active recovery.	Rest/active recovery.	Rest/active recovery.	Rest/active recovery.
TUES	30 min brisk walk.	40 min brisk walk.	30 min easy run.	35 min easy run.	40 min easy run.	5 min easy run, 20 min steady run, 5 min easy run.
WED	Rest.	Rest.	Rest.	Rest.	Rest.	Rest.
THURS	30 min brisk walk.	10 min easy walk, 15 min easy run, 10 min easy walk.	5 min easy run, (3 min hard run, 3 min easy run or walk. Repeat x3), 5 min easy run.	5 min easy run, (4 min hard run, 3 min easy run. Repeat x4), 5 min easy run.	30 min easy run.	5 min easy run, (5 min hard run, 2 min easy run. Repeat x3), 5 min easy run.
FRI	Rest.	Rest.	Rest.	Rest.	Rest	Rest.
SAT/ SUN	10 min steady walk, 20 min easy run, 10 min steady walk.	5 min brisk walk, 25 min easy run, 5 min brisk walk, 5 min easy walk.	40 min easy run.	45 min easy run.	55 min easy run.	60 min easy run.

Half-marathon:
Beginner 12 week schedule

Monday and Saturday or Sunday are rest or active recovery days. Tuesday is for developing race endurance. Wednesday and Friday are rest days. Thursday is for intervals. Your weekend running day is for building strength and stamina.

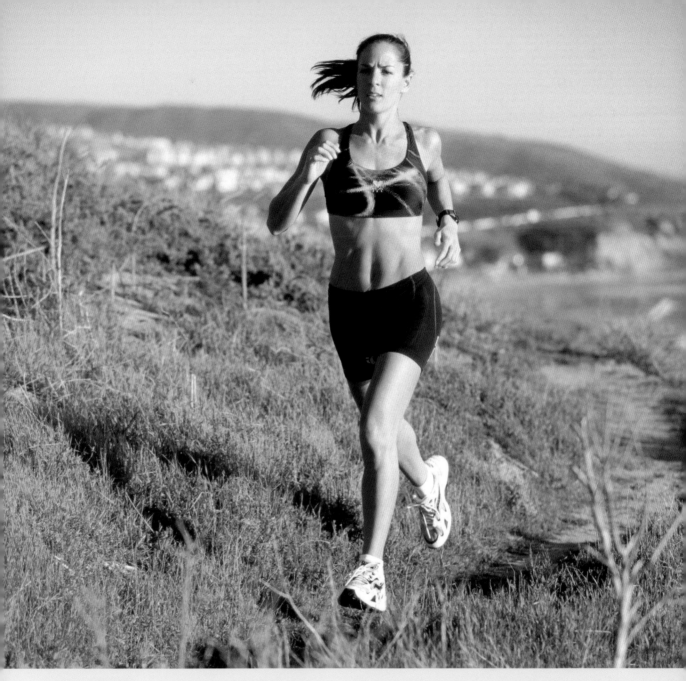

Half-marathon:
Competent 12 week schedule

Monday is a light day. Tuesday builds speed endurance. Wednesday is an active recovery day. Thursday develops race-pace running. Friday is a rest day. Saturday is a steady day and for mixed-pace running. Sunday is for developing strength and stamina; from Week 6, practise your hydration strategy (see page 122) on this day.

	WEEK 1	WEEK 2	WEEK 3	WEEK 4	WEEK 5	WEEK 6
MON	30 min easy run.	30 min easy run.	40 min easy run.	45 min steady run.	30 min steady run.	30 min easy run (am), 20 min easy run (pm).
TUES	30 min easy run.	10 min easy run, (3 min hard run, 2 min easy run. Repeat x4), 10 min easy run.	10 min easy run, (3 min hard run, 2 min easy run. Repeat x6), 10 min easy run.	10 min easy run, (3 min hard run, 1 min easy run. Repeat x6), 10 min easy run.	45 min easy run.	10 min easy run, (5 min hard run, 2 min easy run. Repeat x5), 15 min easy run.
WED	Active recovery.	Active recovery.	Active recovery.	Active recovery.	Active recovery.	Active recovery.
THURS	45 min easy run.	45 min run.	5 min easy run, 20 min tempo, 5 min easy run.	50 min easy run.	10 min easy run, 20 min steady run, 10 min easy run.	50 min easy run.
FRI	Rest.	Rest.	Rest.	Rest.	Rest.	Rest.
SAT	30 min steady run.	10 min easy run, 40 min fartlek, 10 min easy run.	40 min easy run.	10 min easy run, 30 min tempo, 10 min easy run.	50 min easy run.	5 min easy run, 15 min steady run, 15 min hard run, 10 min steady run, 10 min hard run, 5 min easy run.
SUN	60 min easy run.	75 min easy run.	85 min easy run.	75 min easy run.	90 min easy run or RACE 10 km (6.2 miles) with 20 min warm-up/warm-down.	100 min easy run.

	WEEK 7	WEEK 8	WEEK 9	WEEK 10	WEEK 11	WEEK 12
MON	30 min easy run (am), 20 min easy run (pm).	45 min easy run.	Rest.	45 min easy run.	Rest.	Rest.
TUES	10 min easy run, (6 min hard run, 2 min easy run. Repeat x5), 10 min easy run.	10 min easy run, (8 min hard run, 2 min easy run. Repeat x3), 10 min easy run.	10 min easy run, (6 min hard run, 1 min easy run. Repeat x5), 10 min easy run.	10 min easy run, (5 min hard run, 1 min easy run. Repeat x5), 10 min easy run.	5 min easy run, (6 min hard run, 2 min easy run. Repeat x6), 5 min easy run.	5 min easy run, (5 min half-marathon-pace run, 5 min easy run. Repeat x3), 5 min easy run.
WED	Active recovery.	Active recovery.	Active recovery.	Active recovery.	Active recovery.	Active recovery.
THURS	45 min steady run.	45 min steady run.	20 min easy run, 30 min half-marathon-pace run, 10 min easy run.	45 min easy run.	10 min easy run, 25 min half-marathon-pace run, 10 min easy run.	Rest.
FRI	Rest.	Rest.	Rest.	Rest.	Rest.	Rest.
SAT	5 min easy run, 40 min tempo, 5 min easy run.	30 min easy run.	10 min easy run, (3 min hard run, 90 sec easy run. Repeat x3), 5 min easy run, (3 min hard run, 90 sec easy run. Repeat x3), 5 min easy run, (3 min hard run, 90 sec easy run. Repeat x2), 5 min easy run.	10 min run, 20 min steady run, 20 min hard run, 20 min steady run, 5 min easy run.	40 min easy run.	Rest.
SUN	105 min easy run.	110 min steady run.	90 min easy run.	105 min easy run.	75 min easy run.	RACE DAY.

131

Top training tips

Marathon nutrition:
- *During your last week of training, avoid junk food and eat sensibly to fuel up for your race (see pages 28–33).*
- *Make sure you include carbohydrates in your diet on the two days before the race.*
- *Eat a well-balanced diet with plenty of carbohydrates in the week after the race to replace your depleted stores.*

Marathon strategy

- Review your personal and work commitments, and allow sufficient time for your training.
- Practise racing. Run from about 8 km (5 miles) up to half-marathon to test your fitness in the months leading up to the race.
- Set yourself a realistic but challenging target for your race. Work out time splits for this pace and practise running at this speed (see page 101).
- Practise using energy drinks during running (see page 122).
- Don't try anything new (such as running shoes) in the immediate run-up.
- Try to rest in the final few days. The hard work is done, so save your energy!
- For personalized crowd support during the race, print your name on your running vest.
- The middle part of the race will be the most challenging — concentrate hard!
- Use the drinks stations to break up the distance and get you to the finish.
- A minimum of one week with no running is advisable after the race. Light activity, such as walking, will promote recovery.

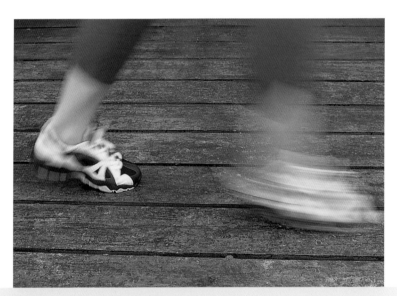

Running a marathon

You have taken a big step in deciding to run a marathon. This is a demanding event that requires careful planning and preparation. In reality, training should start a few months (ideally four to six) before the race date. Those who are well prepared and ready for the challenge will reach the finish faster and in better physical condition than someone who has significantly underestimated the effort required.

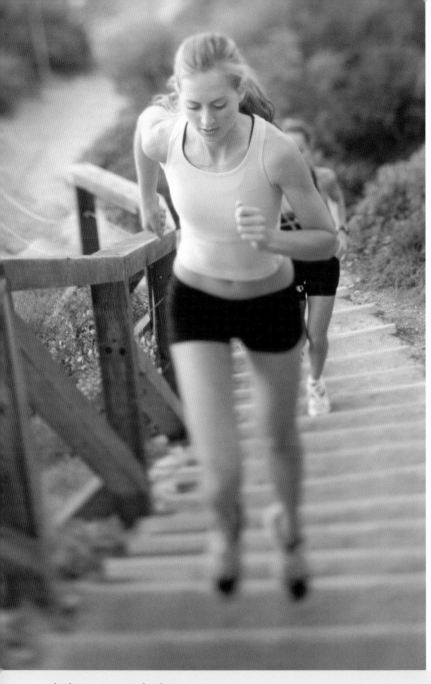

Monday and Friday are rest days. Tuesday is for steady-paced running. Wednesday and Saturday or Sunday are active recovery days – take time to stretch and maybe swim. Thursday is for mixed-paced efforts. Your weekend running day is for building strength, stamina and your long run, and for practising your hydration strategy (see page 122). From Week 9, wear your race-day kit to make sure it is comfortable. Start tapering your training volume from Week 10.

Marathon:
Beginner 12 week schedule

Once you have attained a basic level of running fitness, it takes a further *minimum* of 12 weeks to prepare appropriately for a marathon. This beginners' marathon schedule assumes that you have a little running experience and have steadily built up your running so that you can confidently keep going without stopping for 30 minutes of easy running (see the training schedules on pages 79 and 81–82).

	WEEK 1	WEEK 2	WEEK 3	WEEK 4	WEEK 5	WEEK 6
MON	Rest.	Rest.	Rest.	Rest.	Rest.	Rest.
TUES	30 min steady walk.	40 min brisk walk.	10 min easy walk, 20 min easy run, 10 min easy walk.	35 min easy run.	15 min steady run, (3 min hard run, 1 min walk. Repeat x6), 15 min easy run.	30 min steady run.
WED	Active recovery.	Active recovery.	Active recovery.	Active recovery.	Active recovery.	Active recovery.
THURS	10 min brisk walk, 20 min easy run, 10 min easy walk.	15 min easy walk, 20 min easy run, 10 min easy walk.	10 min easy run, 10 min steady run, 10 min hard run, 10 min easy run.	10 min easy run, (6 min hard run, 3 min easy run. Repeat x3), 10 min easy run.	30 min easy run.	10 min easy run, (8 min hard run, 2 min easy run. Repeat x3), 10 min easy run.
FRI	Rest.	Rest.	Rest.	Rest.	Rest.	Rest.
SAT/ SUN	15 min steady walk, 30 min easy run, 10 min steady walk.	10 min brisk walk, 45 min easy run, 5 min brisk walk, 5 min easy walk.	5 min brisk walk, 30 min steady run, 5 min brisk walk, 30 min easy walk, 5 min easy walk.	40 min easy run, 5 min easy walk, 40 min easy run.	RACE 10 km (6.2 miles) or up to half-marathon.	(30 min easy run, 5 min walk. Repeat x3.)

	WEEK 7	WEEK 8	WEEK 9	WEEK 10	WEEK 11	WEEK 12
MON	Rest.	Rest.	Rest.	Rest.	Rest.	Rest.
TUES	35 min steady run.	40 min easy run.	40 min easy run.	20 min easy run.	25 min easy run.	5 min easy run, 1.6 km (1 mile) marathon-pace run, 5 min easy run.
WED	Active recovery.	Active recovery.	Active recovery.	Active recovery.	Active recovery.	Active recovery.
THURS	10 min easy run, 10 min steady run, 10 min hard run, 10 min steady run, 10 min easy run.	10 min easy run, 40 min tempo, 10 min easy run.	10 min easy run, (5 min hard run, 2 min easy run. Repeat x4), 10 min easy run.	10 min easy run, 30 min marathon-pace run, 10 min easy run.	5 min easy run, (30 sec hard run, 30 sec easy walk. Repeat x4), 5 min easy run.	10 min very easy run.
FRI	Rest.	Rest.	Rest.	Rest.	Rest.	Rest.
SAT/ SUN	(30 min easy run, 3 min easy walk. Repeat x4).	5 min brisk walk, 60 min easy run, 5 min brisk walk, 60 min easy run, 10 min brisk walk. Focus hard.	5 min brisk walk, 75 min easy run, 5 min easy walk, 45 min easy run, 5 min easy walk, 30 min easy run.	90 min easy run.	60 min easy run.	Sat: Rest. Sun: RACE DAY.

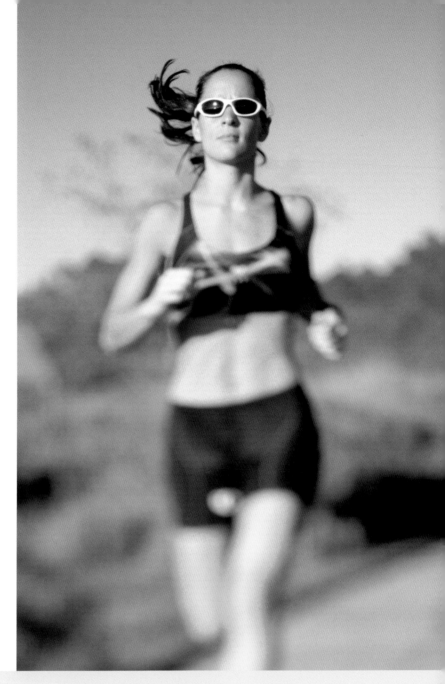

Monday is a light day. Tuesday is for building base stamina through steady running. Wednesday and Saturday or Sunday are rest or active recovery days. Thursday is for mixed-pace running to help with faster running. Friday is a rest day. Your weekend running day is for your long run, developing your endurance and practising your hydration strategy (see page 122). From Week 9, wear your kit on this day, to make sure it is comfortable. Start tapering the volume of your training from Week 10.

Marathon:
Improver 12 week schedule

Improvers should be able to run for an hour without stopping or should have completed a 10 km (6.2 mile) and/or a half-marathon event before starting on this marathon schedule. If you are uncertain about commencing, first complete the beginners' 10 week schedule on pages 81–82.

	WEEK 1	WEEK 2	WEEK 3	WEEK 4	WEEK 5	WEEK 6
MON	20 min easy run.	25 min easy run.	30 min easy run.	30 min easy run.	Rest.	Rest.
TUES	40 min easy run.	40 min steady run.	40 min steady run.	10 min easy run, 30 min tempo, 10 min easy run.	10 min easy run, (30 sec hard run, 1 min easy run. Repeat x4), 10 min easy run.	45 min easy run.
WED	Rest/active recovery.	Rest/active recovery.	Rest/active recovery.	Rest/active recovery.	Rest/active recovery.	Rest/active recovery.
THURS	10 min easy run, 20 min steady run, 10 min easy run.	10 min easy run, 30 min fartlek, 10 min easy run.	5 min easy run, 20 min steady run, 10 min hard run, 5 min easy run.	10 min easy run, (5 min hard run, 3 min easy run. Repeat x4), 10 min easy run.	30 min steady run.	55 min steady run.
FRI	Rest.	Rest.	Rest.	Rest.	Rest.	Rest.
SAT/ SUN	60 min easy run.	75 min easy run.	90 min easy run.	105 min easy run.	RACE half-marathon.	110 min steady run.

Schedule continues on page 138

	WEEK 7	WEEK 8	WEEK 9	WEEK 10	WEEK 11	WEEK 12
MON	40 min steady run.	30 min easy run.	20 min easy run.	Rest.	Rest.	Rest.
TUES	15 min easy run, 45 min tempo, 15 min easy run.	15 min easy run, 30 min hard run, 5 min easy run, 10 min hard run, 10 min easy run.	15 min easy run, 40 min marathon-pace run, 15 min easy run.	10 min easy run, 30 min steady run, 10 min easy run.	10 min easy run, 20 min marathon-pace run, (1 min hard run, 1 min easy walk. Repeat x4), 10 min easy run.	10 min easy run, 1.6 km (1 mile) run at marathon pace, 10 min easy run, 1.6 km (1 mile) run at marathon race pace, 10 min easy run.
WED	Rest/active recovery.	Rest/active recovery.	Rest/active recovery.	Rest/active recovery.	Rest/active recovery.	Rest.
THURS	10 min easy run, 10 min steady run, 10 min hard run, 10 min steady run, 10 min easy run.	15 min easy run, (5 min hard run, 2 min easy run. Repeat x5), 10 min easy run.	15 min easy run, (8 min hard run, 2 min easy run. Repeat x4), 15 min easy run.	45 min steady run.	30 min easy run.	5 min very easy run, 2x 100 m steady efforts, 5 min easy run.
FRI	Rest.	Rest.	Rest.	Rest.	Rest.	Rest.
SAT/ SUN	2 hr 10 min easy run.	2 hr 30 min easy run.	2 hr 50 min easy run.	90 min easy run.	60 min easy run.	Sat: Rest. Sun: RACE DAY.

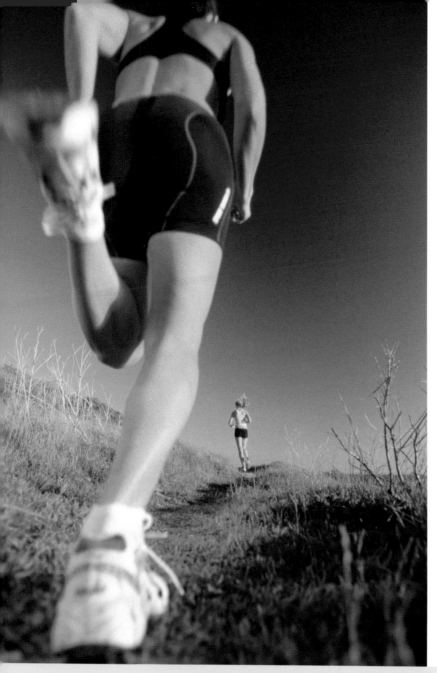

Monday is a light day. Tuesday is an intervals day, for developing speed endurance and threshold running. Wednesday is an active recovery day – go to the gym or for a swim to build core and leg strength. Thursday is for steady running. Friday is a rest day. The weekend is for building stamina and strength to help you go the distance, and for practising your race-day pace and hydration strategies (see page 122). From Week 9, wear your race kit to make sure it is comfortable. Start tapering your training volume from Week 10.

Marathon:
Competent 12 week schedule

Runners should be able to run for an hour without stopping or should have completed a 10 km (6.2 mile) and/or a half-marathon event before starting on this schedule. The competent marathon schedule is for you if you run regularly and have experience of longer-distance running.

	WEEK 1	WEEK 2	WEEK 3	WEEK 4	WEEK 5	WEEK 6
MON	Rest.	Rest.	30 min easy run.	30 min easy run.	30 min easy run.	Rest.
TUES	10 min easy run, 20 min faster run, 10 min easy run.	10 min easy run, (2 min hard run, 90 sec easy run. Repeat x5), 10 min easy run.	15 min easy run, (3 min hard run, 2 min easy run. Repeat x5), 15 min easy run.	15 min easy run, (5 min hard run, 2 min easy run. Repeat x4), 15 min easy run.	20 min easy run, (30 sec hard run, 1 min walk. Repeat x6), 15 min easy run.	20 min easy run, 20 min steady run, 20 min easy run.
WED	Active recovery.	Active recovery.	Active recovery.	Active recovery.	Rest.	Active recovery.
THURS	35 min easy run.	40 min easy run.	45 min easy run.	10 min easy run, 25 min steady run, 10 min easy run.	40 min easy run.	55 min steady run.
FRI	Rest.	Rest.	Rest.	Rest.	Rest.	Rest.
SAT	45 min easy run.	12 min easy run, 40 min quite hard run on hilly circuit if possible, 12 min easy run.	RACE 10 km (6.2 miles) or 10 min easy run, 50 min tempo on a flat course, 10 min easy run.	75 min easy run.	Rest.	10 min easy run, 40 min fartlek, 10 min easy run.
SUN	60 min easy run.	75 min easy run.	90 min easy run.	30 min easy run, 20 min steady run, 20 min easy run, 20 min steady run, 15 min easy run.	RACE half-marathon.	10 min very easy run, 100 min steady run, 10 min easy run.

	WEEK 7	WEEK 8	WEEK 9	WEEK 10	WEEK 11	WEEK 12
MON	25 min easy run.	30 min easy run.	20 min easy run.	Rest.	Rest.	Rest.
TUES	15 min easy run, (6 min hard run, 2 min easy run. Repeat x4), 15 min easy run.	10 min easy run, 30 min tempo, 5 min easy run, 20 min tempo, 10 min easy run.	40 min easy run.	15 min easy run, 30 min hard run, 15 min easy run.	10 min easy run, 20 min marathon-pace run, (1 min hard run, 1 min walk. Repeat x4), 10 min easy.	10 min easy run, 1.6 km (1 mile) run at marathon pace, 10 min easy run, 1.6 km (1 mile) run at marathon pace, 10 min easy run.
WED	Active recovery.	Active recovery.	Active recovery.	Active recovery.	Active recovery.	20 min easy run.
THURS	45 min easy run.	50 min easy run.	15 min easy run, (8 min hard run, 2 min easy run. Repeat x4), 15 min easy run.	45 min steady run.	30 min easy run.	Rest.
FRI	Rest.	Rest.	Rest.	Rest.	Rest.	5 min very easy run including 2x 100 m steady run, 5 min very easy run.
SAT	75 min steady run.	40 min steady run.	10 min easy run, 50 min marathon-pace run, 10 min easy run.	60 min easy run.	Rest.	Rest.
SUN	2 hr 10 min easy run.	2 hr 30 min run including 30 min easy run, 60 min steady run, 30 min easy run, 20 min steady run, 10 min easy run.	2 hr 50 min easy run.	1 hr 40 min steady run.	60 min easy run.	RACE DAY.

Index

Publisher acknowledgements

Executive Editor: Katy Denny
Editor: Fiona Robertson
Executive Art Editor: Karen Sawyer
Designer: Martin Topping @ 'ome Design
Picture Research: Aruna Mathur
Senior Production Controller: Martin Croshaw

Picture acknowledgements

Key: b = bottom; c = centre; l = left; r = right; t = top
ActionPlus/Mike Hewitt 123; /Erik Isakson 80, 129, 133, 136, 139;
/Glyn Kirk 95; /Phillippe Millereau 12–13, 38–39. **Alamy** 42. **Corbis
UK Ltd**/Chris Cole 24; /John Kolesidis 92–93; /William Sallaz 22;
/Pete Saloutos 109. **Getty Images** 94; /Stu Forster 102; /John
Glustina 50; /Fernando Leon 96; /John Terence Turner 40. **Octopus
Publishing Group Limited** 64 b; /Stephen Conroy 30 r; /William
Lingwood 30 l, 32; /Neil Mersh 31 t; /Peter Myers 84, 85; /Lis
Parsons 31 b; /Peter Pugh-Cook 28, 52 l, 52 r, 53 l, 53 r, 54 t, 54 b,
55 t, 55 c, 55 b, 56, 57 l, 57 r, 58 t, 58 b, 59 t, 59 br, 59 bl, 64 t, 65 t,
65 b, 66 t, 66 b, 67 t, 67 b, 68 tl, 68 tr, 68 br, 68 bl, 69 tl, 69 c, 69 tr,
69 br, 69 bl, 70 t, 70 tc, 70 bc, 70 b, 71 tl, 71 tr, 71 br, 71 bl, 72 t, 72
c, 72 b, 73 t, 73 c, 73 b, 74 t, 74 c, 74 b, 75 t, 75 c, 75 b, 76 l, 76 r,
77 l, 77 r, 77 c; /William Reavell 29, 31 c, 88; /Unit Photographic 18;
/Ian Wallace 132.Photodisc 8, 27, 34, 35, 86. **Photolibrary
Group**/Brandx Pictures 60; /Creatas 26, 48; /Florian Franke 9;
/Photoalto 78, 106; /plainpicture 46; /Randy Lincks 19; /Stockbyte
47; /Teo Lannie 14; /Werran/Ochsner 126. *Running fitness*
magazine 7, 15, 16, 20, 25, 43, 44, 62, 83, 89, 100, 104, 105,
122.www.running4women.com 98.

Author acknowledgements

This book would not have been possible without the help and
support I have received from a number of people. Thank you to
Katy Denny and Hamlyn for giving me the opportunity to inspire
and encourage women to take up a sport I love and get so much
from. Thanks also to Paul Larkins at *Running fitness*, to my mum for
being brave enough to take me running as a child, and to my running
coaches of the past 21 years, Alex and Rosemary Stanton. Alex has
been a rock throughout my life as well as in my athletics career. He
has inspired me to strive for great heights and we continue to aim
for the goals I have yet to achieve. I owe him so much. I would also
like to thank my husband, Martin, who has given me all the support,
stability and encouragement that I have demanded over the last
twelve years and has undoubtedly contributed to my athletic
success. His contributions have been instrumental in writing this
guide to women's running, and our experiences and lives together
have also served to inform its shape and contents.

If you have been inspired by this book and would like
further support with your running or a personal training
programme, then you can contact Liz Yelling at her website
www.active-futures.com. There are also many other online
running communities where you can find encouragement and
information, including **www.running4women.com**, the
fastest-growing website for women runners in the world.

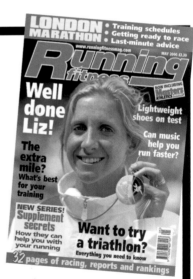